MAKING SENSE of the
Chest X-ray

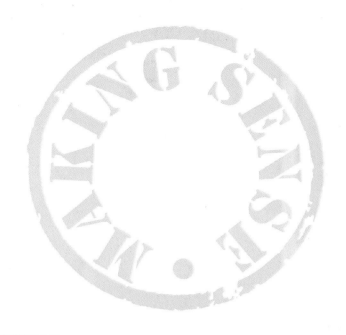

MAKING SENSE of the
Chest X-ray
A hands-on guide

Second edition

Paul F. Jenkins
Formerly Winthrop Professor of Acute
Medicine at the University of Western
Australia
and
Consultant Physician, Norfolk and Norwich
University Hospital

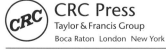

CRC Press
Taylor & Francis Group
Boca Raton London New York

CRC Press is an imprint of the
Taylor & Francis Group, an **informa** business

CRC Press
Taylor & Francis Group
6000 Broken Sound Parkway NW, Suite 300
Boca Raton, FL 33487-2742

© 2013 by Taylor & Francis Group, LLC
CRC Press is an imprint of Taylor & Francis Group, an Informa business

No claim to original U.S. Government works

Printed and bound in India by Replika Press Pvt. Ltd.
Version Date: 20121126

International Standard Book Number: 978-1-4441-3515-2 (Paperback)

Visit the Taylor & Francis Web site at
http://www.taylorandfrancis.com

and the CRC Press Web site at
http://www.crcpress.com

Contents

Preface

This book is intended as a practical guide for doctors and other healthcare professionals who need to interpret a chest X-ray comprehensively and competently as part of their overall assessment of sick patients. The chest radiograph is an immensely valuable tool and proficiency in its interpretation is a fundamental skill for physicians. Despite this, my experience has been that clinical doctors are rarely taught practical radiographic techniques and chest X-ray abnormalities are commonly missed or incorrectly diagnosed as a result.

The book does not provide an exhaustive reference for differential diagnosis based on the chest X-ray – standard radiology texts exist for this purpose – but, rather, is intended to engender an accurate and comprehensive approach to radiographic interpretation by stressing the need for a systematic approach to analysis. Throughout the book, a problem-solving approach to interpretation is emphasized; if an abnormality is seen, a sequence of questions is set in train with an active search for supplementary radiographic signs that might allow a definitive diagnosis – a proactive, systematic approach is far more efficient and less likely to miss diagnostic radiographic clues.

For example, a chest X-ray showing consolidation in the right mid-zone should provoke a sequence of active questioning as follows:

- How well circumscribed is the shadowing?
- How dense is it (soft tissue or denser)?
- Is there an air-bronchogram within it?
- Is cavitation present?
- Does significant loss of volume accompany the consolidated lung?
- Is there associated pleural disease, bone disease or lymphadenopathy?

A successful problem-solving approach relies on knowing which questions to ask and I have tried to address this in the chapters that follow. If, in the example of consolidation quoted above, further analysis should reveal significant loss of volume in the consolidated lobe, with an absent air-bronchogram, concerns about proximal bronchial obstruction and perhaps bronchial carcinoma would be heightened, prompting urgent further investigation. Alternative diagnostic implications would accrue if cavitation were observed in the area of consolidation. Specific infective causes of pneumonia, including *Staphylococcus*, tuberculosis and Gram-negative organisms then enter the differential diagnosis as well as non-infective pathologies such as vasculitis. In any case, clinical concerns would be heightened, further investigations would be mandatory and management would be facilitated by comprehensive radiographic interpretation.

Another example is illustrated by the X-ray in Fig. 1, showing an alveolar-filling pattern in the mid-zones, which seems to be perihilar in distribution. The differential diagnosis here is wide and includes pulmonary oedema, pulmonary alveolar haemorrhage, adult respiratory distress syndrome and pneumonia – in fact, any pathological process that can result in alveolar filling should be considered. However, further, proactive analysis reveals additional diagnostic clues with a small right pleural effusion, cardiomegaly and septal lines at the bases (illustrated in Fig. 2). With this combination of features, one can be confident of the diagnosis of heart failure and the presence of sternal sutures provides additional evidence of heart disease.

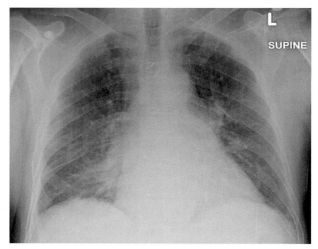

Figure 1

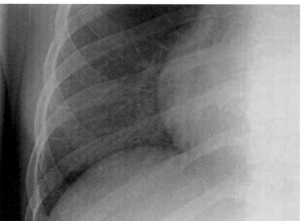

Figure 2

The diagnostic usefulness of a chest X-ray is enhanced tremendously when combined with knowledge of the clinical findings and a 'collaborative' diagnostic approach is encouraged throughout the book, with a 'clinical connections' icon (⊚) to emphasize the partnership.

Icons are also used to highlight potential hazards (⚡), interesting facts or 'pearls of wisdom' (◉) and topics that link the other chapters (⊗).

Finally, I have chosen illustrations that show more than one abnormality. This is intentional in order to emphasize a fundamental theme of the book, namely the need for obsessional, systematic interpretation of the chest X-ray. A sequence of analysis must be adhered to in order to assimilate all of the information the radiograph has to offer.

Finding an abnormality must not call a halt to analysis. Rather, it should stimulate a systematic search for additional abnormal findings that will assist in narrowing the differential diagnosis – in this way, safe and effective patient management will be optimized.

Acknowledgements

Much of the discussion in this book has evolved from the 'problem-solving' teaching sessions I have led over the years and I am deeply indebted to those whom I have taught – I have learnt so much from them.

The team at Hodder has been superb and I extend especial thanks to Joanna Koster, Jenny Wright and Joanna Silman for their help, forbearance and professionalism.

I was gently guided towards medical studies by my parents, Ioan and Betty Jenkins and I could never thank them enough. This book is dedicated to them and to my wife, Glynis, my two sons, David and Peter and to my lovely daughters-in-law, Janelle and Polly with thanks for their support, advice, love and friendship.

List of abbreviations

AP	antero-posterior
CT	computed tomography
CTPA	computed tomography pulmonary angiogram
F_IO_2	inspired oxygen concentration
PA	postero-anterior
P_ACO_2	alveolar carbon dioxide tension
P_aCO_2	arterial carbon dioxide tension
P_aO_2	arterial oxygen tension
P_AO_2	alveolar oxygen tension
P_IO_2	inspired oxygen tension
S_aO_2	arterial oxygen saturation
V_A	alveolar ventilation

CHAPTER 1

The systematic approach

There are two basic elements to the systematic interpretation of a chest radiograph. The first is the structure of the system itself and this chapter describes the sequence of interpretation I have developed over the years. Whether you adopt this system or develop your own, it is essential to be disciplined and not deviate from a structured approach. Train yourself to examine anatomical structures in strict order because deviation will risk missing important information. A classic example is your eye being drawn to an obvious abnormality. You note the abnormality and it is easy to consider 'job done' ignoring further critical examination. This happened recently when a radiographic diagnosis was considered complete after multiple rounded shadows were detected in the lung fields. These were well defined, variable in size and clearly represented metastatic malignant disease. Unfortunately, the right mastectomy, readily visible on the radiograph and the likely source of the metastatic deposits, was missed and this was simply because the breast shadows were not examined specifically as part of a systematic approach. I have known osteolytic lesions in ribs (accompanying an obvious lung mass) to be missed for exactly the same reason. So, develop a sequential system of observation and do not deviate from it.

The second element is to 'problem-solve' as you follow your systematic interpretation. By this I mean ask specific questions at each stage of the examination. Is an anatomical structure of normal size, is it correctly positioned and are its borders well defined? What are the detailed features of any pulmonary infiltrate – distribution, size and shape of component shadows, presence of calcification and so on? In other words, go in search of information and do not just wait for it to hit you in the eye – this is a basic, generic skill of clinical medicine.

There is a third element that will accrue with experience and this is 'pattern recognition' – an ability to recognize heart failure because you have seen the pattern hundreds of times and recognize it. Pattern recognition is another generic skill of the art of clinical medicine and should not be disparaged but use it warily and do not allow yourself to abbreviate the systematic approach – even the most experienced of us has been caught out by ignoring this fundamental maxim.

Here is the system I follow.

BASIC OBSERVATIONS FIRST

- Note the patient's name, age and ethnic background. These details may provide clues to the possible diagnosis.
- What is the date of the radiograph? A stunning radiographic diagnosis is far more relevant to patient care if the X-ray is current rather than 2 years old.
- Has the radiograph been taken in postero-anterior (PA) or antero-posterior (AP) projection? If the latter, then it is impossible to comment accurately on heart size.
- How centred is the image? Look at the sterno-clavicular joints when making this assessment. The right and left sterno-clavicular joints are equidistant from the

mid-line in the normal chest X-ray shown in Fig. 1.1 (arrowed) and this is a well-centred radiograph. A rotated film will distort the appearance of all anatomical structures, particularly those within the mediastinum, and interpretation may be impossible if the image is significantly skewed.

- Next, decide on the degree of radiological penetration of the image. Ideal penetration applies when you can see vertebral bodies clearly through the heart shadow. Sometimes a softer film helps in defining pulmonary infiltration and, in these days of digital images, it is possible to manipulate the window level in order to optimize penetration. Figure 1.1 is an example of near-perfect X-ray penetration.

- Finally, examine the alignment of the ribs. In Fig. 1.2 the ribs are horizontal with the anterior and posterior parts of each rib shadow virtually overlying one another. This is an AP X-ray that has been taken with the patient lying back rather than sitting (lordotic). The mediastinum and the hemidiaphragms are very distorted and interpretation is unreliable, a situation exacerbated by the fact that the film is significantly underpenetrated.

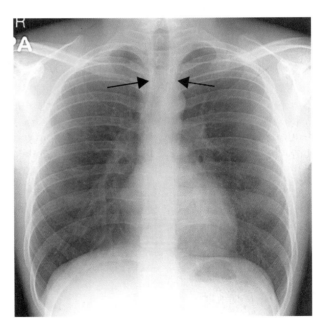

Figure 1.1 Normal chest X-ray.

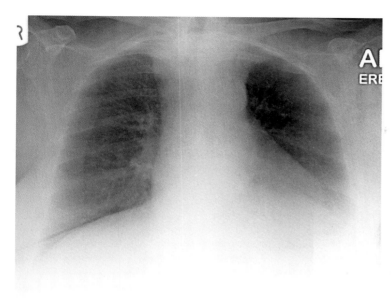

Figure 1.2 An underpenetrated lordotic chest X-ray. The horizontal appearance of the ribs is the clue to imperfect patient positioning.

PEARLS OF WISDOM

Accurate radiographic interpretation is reliant upon the quality of the X-ray. It is vital to assess penetration, centring and position of the patient before drawing conclusions from the radiographic appearances.

Figure 1.3 illustrates the characteristic acute angle between posterior and lateral ribs in a patient with pectus excavatum. Note the 'fuzziness' adjacent to the right heart border, which is a normal accompaniment of this anatomical variant. Recognition of

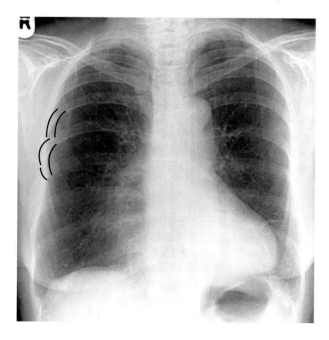

Figure 1.3 The characteristic acute angle between posterior and lateral ribs (highlighted) in a patient with pectus excavatum. Note the shadowing adjacent to the right heart border, which is a normal association of this chest wall shape.

pectus excavatum from the shape of the rib cage will remove the concern that there might be right middle lobe consolidation. Figure 1.4 is a lateral chest X-ray of the same patient, clearly showing the chest wall deformity.

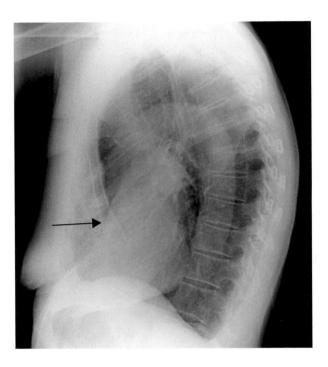

Figure 1.4 A right lateral chest X-ray of the same patient showing the anterior chest wall depression (arrowed).

You are now ready to examine specific areas. 'Problem-solve' as you proceed with critical analysis of areas and anatomical structures in turn, continually asking questions of the appearances you detect.

COMMENCE IN THE NECK

- Is the trachea deviated or compressed? If so, this is compatible with retrosternal thyroid enlargement (Fig. 1.5).
- Can you see surgical emphysema in the soft tissues of the neck? Figure 1.6 is an obvious example in a young person with an acute attack of asthma but the appearances are often subtle and will be missed unless you look for them specifically.

Interestingly, one cannot see a pneumomediastinum in Fig. 1.6, although presumably there is one. Figure 1.7, on the other hand, shows obvious air in the mediastinum in association with a right-sided tension pneumothorax. Once again, surgical emphysema is present in the neck. The combination of pneumomediastinum and pneumothorax must raise the possibility of oesophageal rupture although, in this case, air had leaked from a ruptured bulla into both the pleural cavity and the mediastinum as a complication of acute asthma.

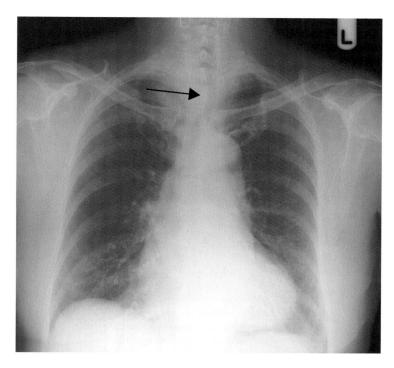

Figure 1.5 Retrosternal thyroid goitre showing indentation and deviation of the trachea (arrowed).

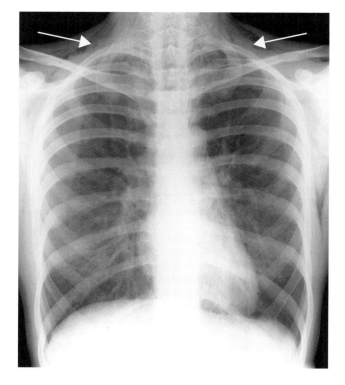

Figure 1.6 Surgical emphysema in the soft tissues of the neck (arrowed), complicating acute asthma.

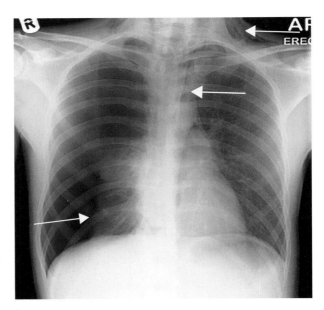

Figure 1.7 Pneumothorax and pneumomediastinum. Note the black line defining the left mediastinal structures, the border of the collapsed right lung and air in the soft tissues of the neck (all arrowed).

HAZARD

It is important to diagnose pneumomediastinum. Asthmatics rarely come to harm from this complication of acute asthma but air in the mediastinum can also result from oesophageal rupture and this condition must not be missed. Spontaneous rupture of the oesophagus does happen. It is usually associated with vomiting but the severity of the vomiting can be surprisingly slight.

CLINICAL CONNECTIONS

The classical physical signs of pneumomediastinum are palpable surgical emphysema in the neck and Hamman's sound. This is a crunching noise heard over the praecordium throughout the cardiac cycle. It is similar to, though more 'crackly' than, a pericardial rub.

- Is there calcification in the area of the thyroid gland, typical of a thyroid adenoma?
- Are cervical ribs present (Fig. 1.8)? These can be responsible for neurological symptoms due to nerve entrapment.

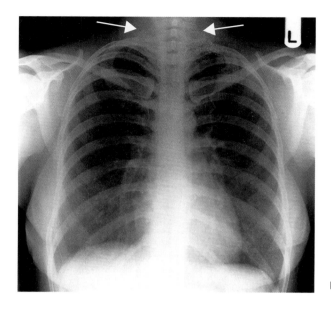

Figure 1.8 Cervical ribs (arrowed).

PROCEED TO THE MEDIASTINUM

Figure 1.9 summarizes the mediastinal structures to be examined. I start with the aortic root.

- Is the aortic root of normal size? If it is small, this may indicate an atrial septal defect and you should seek (proactive 'problem-solving') the ancillary radiographic appearances of this diagnosis – namely, prominent hilar shadows and exaggerated vascular markings in the lung fields (Figs 1.9 and 1.10).

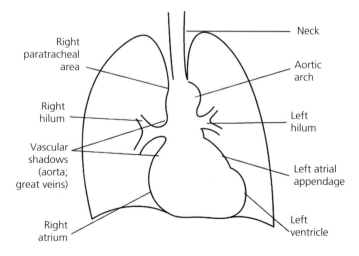

Figure 1.9 Diagram of the mediastinal structures to examine on PA chest X-ray.

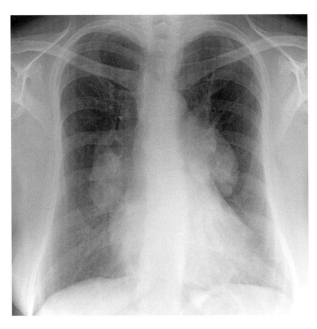

Figure 1.10 Atrial septal defect. This deeply cyanosed 45-year-old woman had an undiagnosed atrial septal defect. On her chest X-ray, the aortic knuckle is small and the hilar shadows are huge. The pulmonary vasculature is prominent proximally but is 'pruned' (i.e. tails out) distally into the lung fields and this indicates established pulmonary hypertension. Unfortunately, because the left-to-right intracardiac shunt had gone undiagnosed for many years, it had resulted in pulmonary hypertension and the shunt had reversed to become 'right-to-left'. In other words, this is an example of Eisenmenger's syndrome.

CLINICAL CONNECTIONS

 Clinical confirmation of an atrial septal defect relies on the classical physical signs of a pulmonary flow murmur, a fixed and split second heart sound and a flow murmur in mid-diastole across the tricuspid valve.

- If the aortic root is prominent, the commonest reasons are hypertension or degenerative unfolding of the aorta. Prominence may be associated with thoracic aortic dissection and, although the appearance is uncommon, always look for a 'double-shadow' within a prominent aortic arch. Be aware though that the chest X-ray in aortic dissection is usually normal (see Hazard and Fig. 1.11).

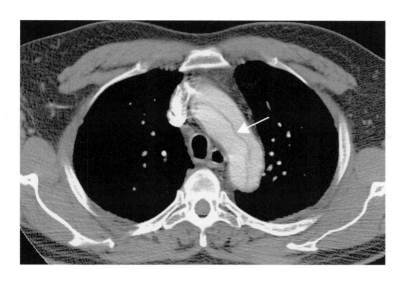

Figure 1.11 Aortic dissection on CT scan – the intimal flap separating the aortic lumen from the dissection is arrowed. The chest X-ray was normal.

⚡ HAZARD

A normal aortic arch on chest X-ray does not exclude aortic dissection. If this diagnosis is suspected computed tomography (CT) (Fig. 1.11) and/or transoesophageal echocardiography is mandatory.

CLINICAL CONNECTIONS

Aortic dissection should be suspected if chest pain is described as tearing in nature, of sudden onset and, especially, if it is felt predominantly in the back.

Now move down the left mediastinal border, analysing as follows:

- Is the left hilum of normal size and shape and in the correct position? The left hilum should be slightly higher than the right on PA view (see Fig. 1.9) and any change in position of either is suggestive of loss of volume in the respective lung field. For example, upward 'shift' of the left hilum is a cardinal feature of loss of volume in left upper lobe and the bilateral upper zone fibrosis of post-primary tuberculosis is associated with upward shift of both hilar shadows (Fig. 1.12).

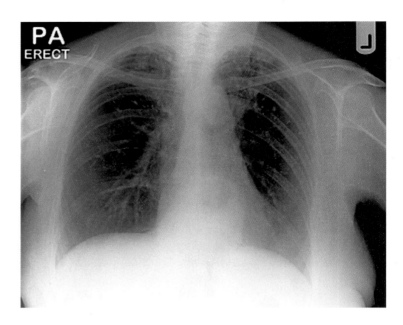

Figure 1.12 Bilateral upward hilar 'shift' as a result of tuberculosis.

LINKS

The concept of 'shift of normal structures' in identifying areas of pulmonary collapse is expanded in Chapter 4.

Deciding whether a hilum is normal or enlarged and, if enlarged, whether the enlargement is due to exaggerated pulmonary vessels or hilar lymphadenopathy is not easy. However, knowledge of a few basic facts and following a systematic approach helps tremendously and this is discussed further in Chapter 2.

- Just below the left hilum is the area, which, if prominent, suggests enlargement of the left atrial appendage as part of left atrial enlargement. This is virtually diagnostic of mitral valve disease and was more commonly seen in the days when rheumatic heart disease was prevalent (Fig. 1.13). To confirm left atrial enlargement, look for the associated widening of the angle of the main carina. The carina forms the superior reflection of the left atrium and becomes 'splayed' if this heart chamber is enlarged.

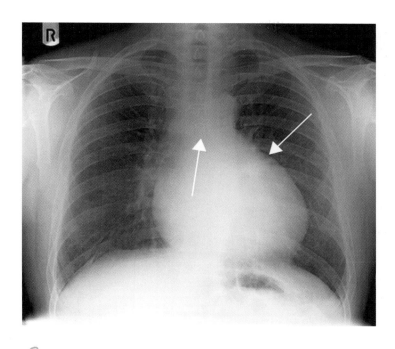

Figure 1.13 Left atrial enlargement; note the prominence of the left atrial appendage and 'splaying' of the main carina, which are both arrowed.

CLINICAL CONNECTIONS

If left atrial enlargement is seen on chest X-ray, listen carefully for the murmurs of mitral valve disease.

- Continue by examining the left ventricular contour. Cardiomegaly is indicative of ventricular dilatation associated with volume overload (aortic or mitral valve regurgitation), primary left ventricular disease (ischaemic or due to a cardiomyopathy) or pericardial effusion (Figs 1.14 and 1.15).

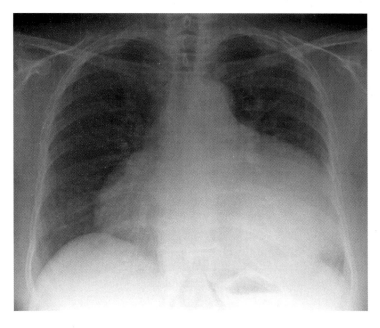

Figure 1.14 Massive cardiomegaly as a result of pericardial effusion.

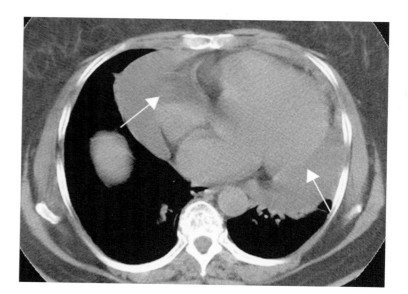

Figure 1.15 CT appearances in the same patient; the pericardial fluid is arrowed.

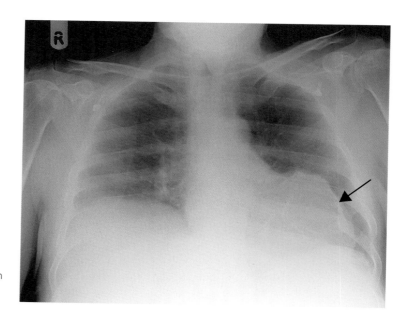

Figure 1.16 A rim of calcification in the wall of a left ventricular aneurysm complicating an old myocardial infarction.

- Calcification can occasionally be seen in the outline of the left ventricle. This is usually indicative of previous myocardial infarction with or without aneurysm formation (Fig. 1.16), although similar calcification can occur in the pericardium as a complication of tuberculosis or with a calcified asbestos pericardial plaque (see Fig. 1.18).
- Now turn your attention to the right mediastinal structures, starting with the right heart border. This normally represents the right atrial shadow and if it is enlarged to the right may suggest tricuspid regurgitation.

CLINICAL CONNECTIONS

The clinical signs of tricuspid regurgitation are:

- 'V' waves (or, more strictly, 'S' systolic waves) in the neck
- an expansile liver
- a pansystolic murmur, heard best at the left sternal edge but often fairly unimpressive.

- The right heart border continues with the ascending aorta, abnormal prominence of which occurs as a result of degenerative unfolding as well as with aneurysm formation.
- Is the right hilum normally positioned and of normal size?
- Examine the paratracheal area. In sarcoidosis, right paratracheal lymphadenopathy is characteristically associated with right hilar enlargement, plus or minus left hilar enlargement (Fig. 1.17).

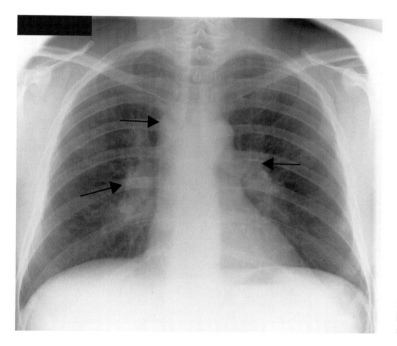

Figure 1.17 Right paratracheal and bilateral hilar lymphadenopathy in sarcoidosis.

You have now successfully completed the 'Mediastinal Circuit'! There is much more regarding specific mediastinal pathology in Chapter 2.

NOW TURN YOUR ATTENTION TO THE PLEURAL REFLECTIONS

Examine each hemidiaphragm in turn and work your way laterally and upwards to each lung apex. Look carefully and ask specific questions; for example, it is so easy to miss calcified asbestos pleural plaques on the hemidiaphragms unless you look for them specifically (Fig. 1.18).

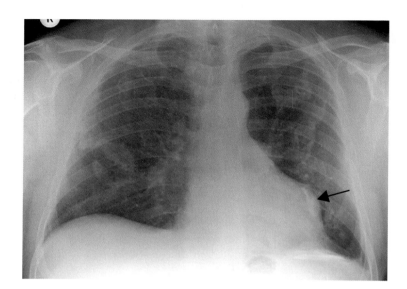

Figure 1.18 Calcified asbestos pleural plaque on left hemidiaphragm. A calcified pericardial plaque can also be seen (arrowed).

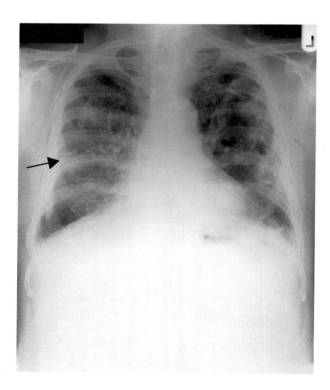

Figure 1.19 'Holly-leaf' pattern of calcified asbestos plaques.

Figure 1.18 also shows the characteristic pleural calcification of asbestos plaques overlying right and left lung fields. This is the so-called 'holly-leaf' pattern. Another example is shown in Fig. 1.19, where a heavily calcified lateral plaque that is following the line of the ribs is arrowed.

THE PENULTIMATE STEP IN YOUR CIRCUIT IS TO CONCENTRATE ON THE LUNG FIELDS

Examine and compare the right and left lung apices, the upper zones, mid-zones and lower zones in turn. Look specifically for:

- differences in density
- the possibility of pulmonary infiltration
- evidence of an alveolar-filling process.

LINKS

How to recognize, differentiate and define a pulmonary infiltrate is covered in detail in subsequent chapters.

Always do your best to explain visible lines. A line in the right mid-zone may indicate a thickened or fluid-filled horizontal fissure. If there is loss of volume in the right lower lobe, the right oblique fissure may become visible as the shrinking lobe moves posteriorly and medially, twisting the oblique fissure around until it is in line with the X-ray beam and then becomes visible. Figure 1.20 shows these and other changes in diagrammatic form.

A peripheral line may indicate a pneumothorax (Fig. 1.21) and a line parallel to part of the mediastinum may be the only clue to the presence of a pneumomediastinum

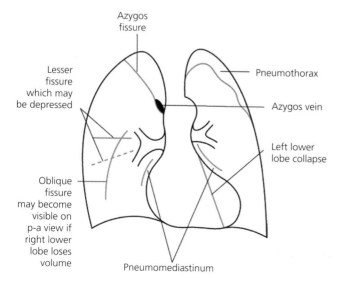

Azygos fissure

Lesser fissure which may be depressed

Oblique fissure may become visible on p-a view if right lower lobe loses volume

Pneumothorax

Azygos vein

Left lower lobe collapse

Pneumomediastinum

Figure 1.20 Common 'lines' on a chest X-ray.

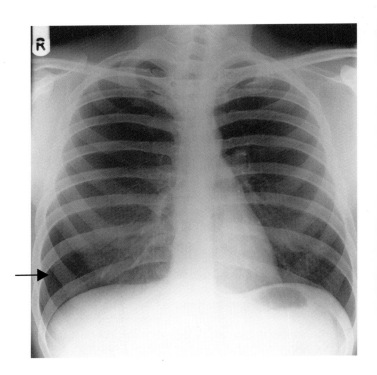

Figure 1.21 Right-sided pneumothorax in a young man. The edge of the lung is arrowed.

(see Fig. 1.7, page 6). Figures 1.22 and 1.23 are examples of other lines that require explanation. Sometimes the appearances are very subtle (Fig. 1.24).

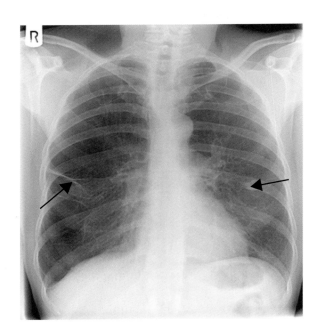

Figure 1.22 Emphysematous bulla in a 44-year-old smoker. There is also a granuloma in the left mid-zone (both arrowed).

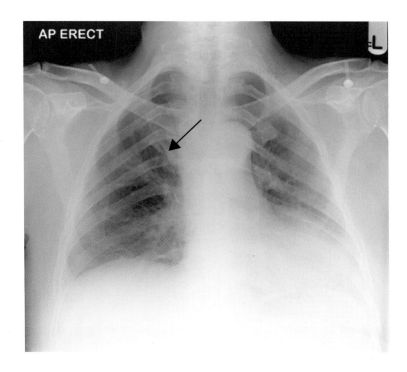

Figure 1.23 The characteristic appearance of an azygos lobe, with the lozenge-shaped azygos vein at its inferior extremity (arrowed).

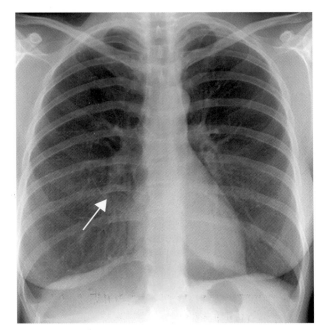

Figure 1.24 Subtle line shadow outlining an emphysematous bulla.

YOU HAVE NOT QUITE FINISHED

It is good discipline to finish by examining four areas specifically. Four areas that are easy to overlook – the 'four Bs', highlighted below.

Behind the heart

Be sure not to miss a hiatus hernia. The enormous incarcerated hiatus hernia shown in Fig. 1.25 is obvious but others may not be and will be missed unless looked for specifically. The clue to other oesophageal pathologies, for example achalasia, may also be found behind the heart with unexplained air/fluid levels.

Look for the tell-tale line of left lower lobe collapse (Fig. 1.26) and, if you think you see it, look specifically for ancillary radiographic signs of collapse (see Chapter 3). Masses behind the heart are easy to overlook. Figure 1.27 shows a neural tumour hiding behind the heart shadow. It is difficult to see on X-ray but the subsequent CT scan was strikingly abnormal (Fig. 1.28).

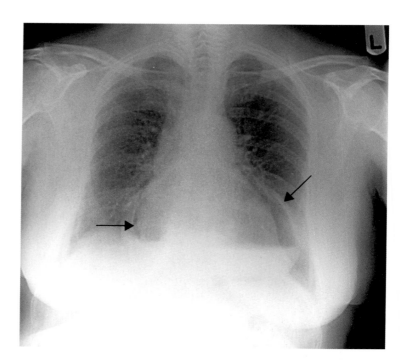

Figure 1.25 Massive hiatus hernia (arrowed).

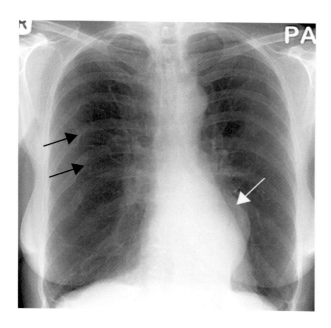

Figure 1.26 Left lower lobe collapse with the responsible bronchial carcinoma arrowed as an obvious mass. Note the old fractures of the right ribs (also arrowed). These were unrelated and had followed a nasty fall some years previously.

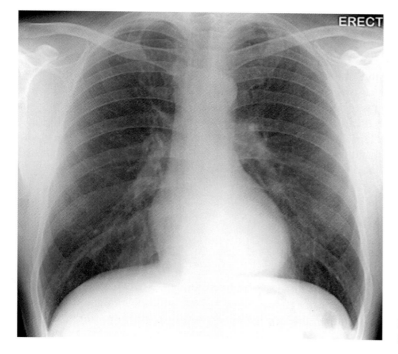

Figure 1.27 Neurogenic tumour posterior to the heart.

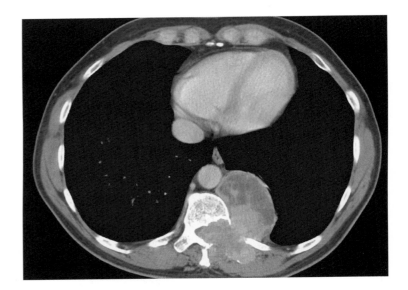

Figure 1.28 CT scan of the patient shown in Fig. 1.27. The tumour can be seen exiting a vertebral foramen (and destroying it in the process). Unhappily, this was a malignant peripheral nerve sheath tumour.

Breast shadows

It is so easy to miss a mastectomy unless you look at the breast shadows specifically. In Fig. 1.29, the eye is drawn to the abnormal parenchymal shadowing in both lung fields but a comprehensive, systematic interpretive approach ensures that the right mastectomy is not missed. The obvious concern was that the lung shadowing was due to metastatic disease but, fortunately, lung biopsy showed changes of cryptogenic organizing pneumonitis, which cleared completely with corticosteroid therapy.

Figure 1.30 is more subtle; both breasts are present but they are very different in shape. It is also possible to see the images of metal clips in the right axilla, which are give-away signs of surgery – in this case lymph node clearance. This woman has undergone right breast lumpectomy for carcinoma. If you now examine the right lung field you will see the elevated horizontal fissure and right hilum indicative of loss of volume in the right upper lobe. An endobronchial secondary deposit was suspected radiographically and was confirmed at bronchoscopy. Fortunately, the response to radiotherapy was good and she was fit and well several years after treatment.

Below the diaphragm

Look specifically for the following:

Air below the diaphragm

Figure 1.31 clearly shows air under the right diaphragm in a young man who had a perforated duodenal ulcer. He was being treated with chemotherapy for non-Hodgkin's lymphoma and right hilar lymphadenopathy is also apparent.

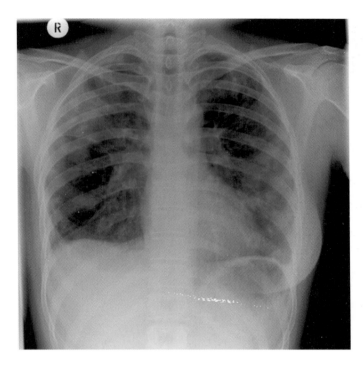

Figure 1.29 Right mastectomy with multiple areas of segmental consolidation in the lung fields, shown on biopsy to be cryptogenic organizing pneumonitis.

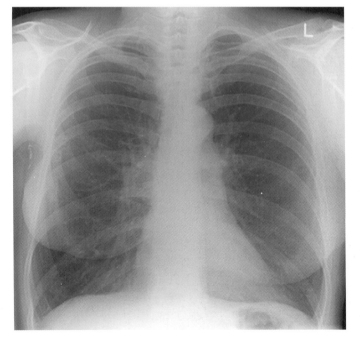

Figure 1.30 Previous lumpectomy of the right breast with metal clips in the right axilla following lymph node clearance. There is also a partial collapse of the right upper lobe, which proved to be due to an endobronchial metastasis from the breast carcinoma.

In Fig. 1.32, there is air below both hemidiaphragms but the appearances are more subtle. This was in a young woman who had undergone laparoscopy for investigation of abdominal pain.

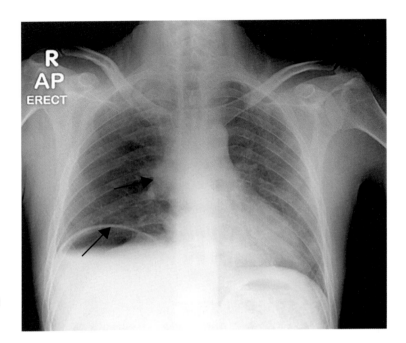

Figure 1.31 Air under the right diaphragm as a result of a perforated duodenal ulcer. Note also the right hilar lymphadenopathy (arrowed).

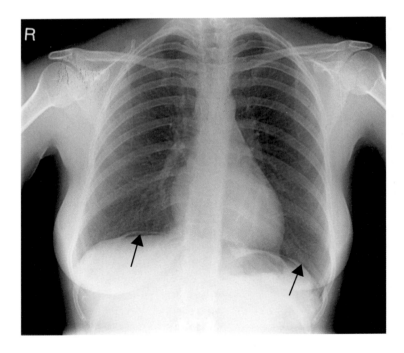

Figure 1.32 Air under both hemidiaphragms (arrowed) following laparoscopy.

Calcification

This is uncommon but calcification within the liver may be due to a hydatid cyst and, within the spleen, is likely to indicate splenic infarction, a recognized complication of sickle cell disease. If the patient's geographic and ethnic origins are known (sheep-rearing areas with hydatid disease or African origin with sickle cell disease) then the diagnosis is secured. I did have examples of both but the films were 'borrowed' I am afraid and I have to settle for an abdominal radiograph showing a calcified hydatid mesenteric cyst in a boy from a hill-farming family in mid-Wales, admitted to a Cardiff hospital when I was a registrar there (Fig. 1.33).

<u>Bones</u>

Look at all bones and joints very carefully – this includes the clavicles, upper arms, and shoulder joints as well as the ribs.

Figure 1.34 shows rib destruction in association with a pancoast tumour of the right lung.

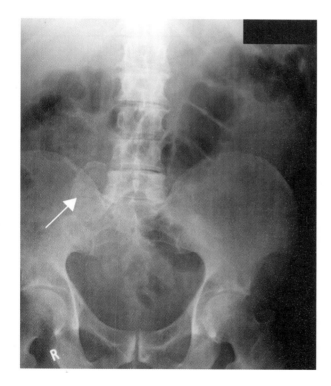

Figure 1.33 The calcified ring shadow of a mesenteric hydatid cyst.

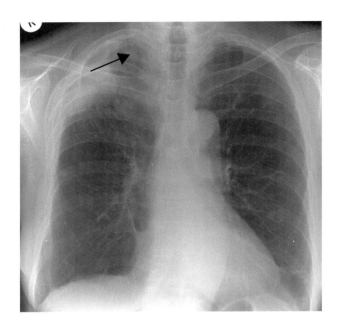

Figure 1.34 Bronchogenic carcinoma of the right upper lobe destroying the right 3rd rib (arrowed).

CLINICAL CONNECTIONS

The patient whose X-ray is shown in Fig. 1.34 had a right-sided Horner's syndrome as well as severe pain in the right arm as a result of invasion of the brachial plexus by the tumour.

Figure 1.35 shows generalized sclerosis in ribs, clavicles and upper arms due to metastatic prostatic carcinoma. This man was admitted with abdominal pain and free air can be seen under the right diaphragm (arrowed) due to a perforated gastric ulcer. Multiple abnormalities are present on this radiograph; they are subtle and you will miss them unless you adhere religiously to a systematic approach.

Figure 1.36 shows an enormously expanding lytic lesion in a left rib.

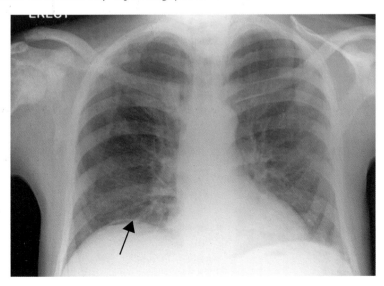

Figure 1.35 Sclerotic bone metastases from prostate cancer.

1 The systematic approach

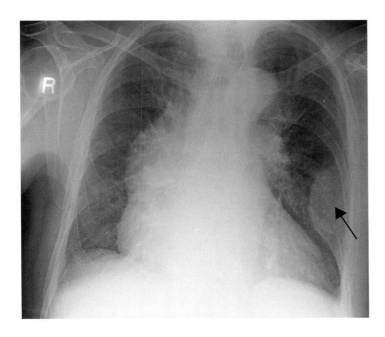

Figure 1.36 This 83-year-old man has an expanding rib lesion on the left as a result of multiple myeloma.

Figure 1.37 shows 'rib-notching' in a young woman who had undergone correction of coarctation of the aorta in childhood. Note the missing left fifth rib, the legacy of her lateral thoracotomy.

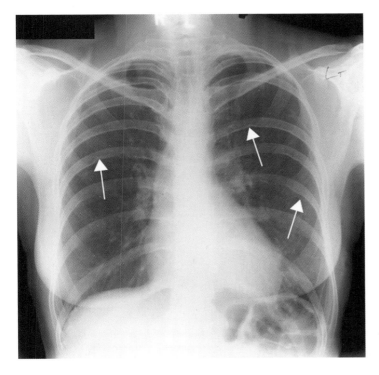

Figure 1.37 Corrected coarctation of the aorta in a young woman. The rib-notching is arrowed (it was much easier to see on the original X-ray) and the left fifth rib is missing following the right lateral thoracotomy.

1 The systematic approach

PEARLS OF WISDOM

It is easier to examine the ribs if you turn the image on its side with the relevant ribs uppermost. Believe me, it really does work!

Finally:

Your systematic examination of the chest radiograph is now complete and it is time to move on to more detailed examination of specific areas.

Check List Chapter 1

✔ Adopt a sequence of analysis and follow it religiously. Don't be diverted from completing your sequence by finding an abnormality and thinking that the job is done.

✔ When you do find an abnormality, glean as much information from it as possible. Do this by asking specific questions, rather than assuming that the information will hit you in the eye. The trick is to know what questions to ask.

✔ If you think you have a diagnosis, seek additional radiographic features to support your hypothesis – for example interstitial lines and pleural effusion(s)v with an infiltrate that you suspect is heart failure.

✔ The system described here (as good as any) is as follows:

- start in the neck
- proceed down the left mediastinum: aortic knuckle, aorto-pulmonary window, left hilum, left atrial appendage, left heart border
- turn to the right heart border and proceed up the right mediastinum to the right hilum and right para-tracheal area
- examine the pleural reflections, starting with the hemidiaphragms
- next is a comprehensive examination of the lung fields.

✔ And, finally, some areas that are easily forgotten and where abnormalities can hide: the 'four Bs'.

CHAPTER 2

The mediastinum and the hila

The mediastinum is a real challenge.

First, radiographic appearances vary considerably in their range of normality here, making it difficult to decide what is normal and what is not.

Second, the mediastinum is a complex structure; abnormalities in specific areas are often subtle and will be missed unless a systematic and sequential approach is adopted as discussed in Chapter 1.

Third, the differential diagnosis of abnormal mediastinal shadowing is diverse and complex.

For these reasons, I like to divide the mediastinum into four 'geographic departments' – superior, anterior, middle and posterior – and combine this with a knowledge of the normal anatomical structures that exist within each. This facilitates a structured approach to the differential diagnosis of abnormal shadowing within each compartment. However, before expanding on this approach, it is useful to consider the hilar shadows separately.

THE 'BULKY' HILUM

There are a few basic points to consider first:

- In a healthy person, the hilar shadows are created by the pulmonary arteries and veins with a small contribution from the major bronchi. The latter appear as narrow line shadows outlined on the one hand by the air contained within them and on the other by adjacent, aerated lung.

- The normal hilar shape is derived from the upper lobe vessels meeting the basal artery and it therefore resembles a letter 'y' lying on its side. The normal shape will be distorted if one limb of the 'y' disappears as a result of collapse of an upper or lower lobe or if additional structures are present, especially abnormal hilar lymph nodes.

- The size of each hilum is best assessed from the size of the respective basal artery, which can usually be identified on a well-penetrated radiograph (Fig. 2.1). The basal artery commonly tapers before it divides into the basal segmental arteries and a convenient and relatively reproducible means of measuring its diameter is at its mid-point. This can be arbitrarily considered to represent the mid-point of the hilum and is the point where the most lateral upper lobe pulmonary vein crosses the basal artery (arrowed). With practice, the lateral upper lobe vein can usually be identified from its typical orientation.

- Starting at the mid-point of the basal artery, measure from its lateral wall to the clearly defined transradiancy of the intermediate bronchus. This is shown in Fig. 2.1 as distance '*a*' and varies in healthy middle-aged adults between 7 and 19 mm with a mean of 14 mm (the measurement '*a*' includes the lateral wall of the intermediate bronchus but this is only about 2 mm and is relatively constant).

The left basal artery is roughly the same size (but commonly 1–2 mm smaller in diameter) when measured at its mid-point, where the most lateral upper lobe vein crosses it (distance '*b*' in Fig. 2.1).

- Quantifying the size of the hilar shadows in this way may seem complicated at first but the exercise becomes much easier with practice and it does add far more objectivity to the assessment of hilar enlargement.

- Clear landmarks are also necessary for identifying the normal position (vertical level on a radiograph) of each hilum. The mid-point of each hilum is identified as described above (arrowed in Fig. 2.1). The mid-point of the right hilum is then opposite the horizontal fissure which meets the sixth rib in the axilla and is also roughly at the level of the third rib anteriorly on deep inspiration. The centre of the left hilum is 0.5–1.5 cm higher. The centre point on each side will be 2–3 cm higher in upper lobe shrinkage and 1–2 cm lower in lower lobe shrinkage.

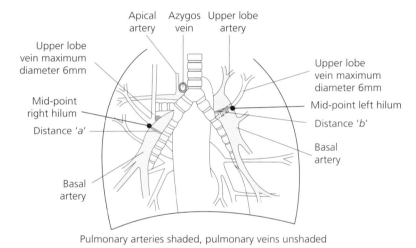

Figure 2.1 Hilar shadows and measurements (see text). '*a*' and '*b*' are diameters measured at the mid-point of the right and left basal artery, respectively. This point is arrowed on each side and is arbitrarily considered to be the mid-point of each hilum. In healthy individuals '*a*' measures 7–19 mm (average 14 mm) and '*b*' is roughly similar though often smaller by 1–2 mm in the same adult.

Pulmonary arteries shaded, pulmonary veins unshaded

PEARL OF WISDOM

A final word regarding normal measurements. Each upper lobe pulmonary vein is 4–6 mm in diameter where it meets its respective basal artery and enlargement occurs in pulmonary venous congestion due to heart failure or mitral valve disease.

- An abnormally prominent hilum is either caused by exaggerated vascular shadowing or by pathological enlargement of non-vascular structures and it is important to attempt to distinguish between the two possibilities. First, the area medial to the mid-point of the right basal artery is the lumen of the intermediate bronchus and it should be radiolucent. Any distortion suggests abnormal pathology, especially lymphadenopathy. Second, identify obvious vascular shadows in the central lung fields and trace them into the hilum. Continue to dissect the hilum in this way and if any component is not obviously vascular in nature, it may well be pathological.

- Although neither of these tips is infallible they do help in deciding if further investigation such as a mediastinal computed tomography (CT) scan is indicated. Figure 2.2 is the chest radiograph of a woman with Eisenmenger's syndrome.

Employing the principles just discussed, we can be confident of the vascular nature of the huge hilar shadows ('*a*' measures 50 mm and '*b*' 45 mm).

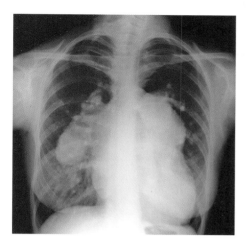

Figure 2.2 Eisenmenger's syndrome with enormous enlargement of the pulmonary vessels.

Figure 2.3 also shows prominent hila due to vascular enlargement. This woman had pulmonary hypertension as a result of chronic obstructive pulmonary disease. Figure 2.4 is an example of bilateral hilar lymphadenopathy in sarcoidosis. Although the medial border of the right basal artery is still outlined, the general 'lumpiness' of both hilar shadows isn't comfortably explained by vascular enlargement. Figure 2.5 emphasizes this point as a more florid example of sarcoid-related bilateral hilar lymphadenopathy.

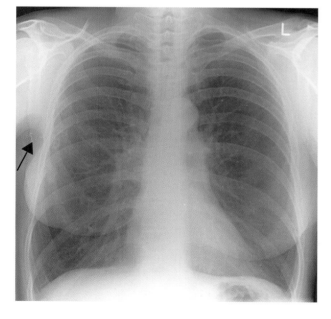

Figure 2.3 Enlargement of proximal pulmonary vessels due to chronic obstructive pulmonary disease in a woman who has had treatment for carcinoma of the right breast. The arrows mark metal clips in the right axilla following axillary lymph node clearance and traumatic fractures of three ribs on the right (see 'Hazard' in the text).

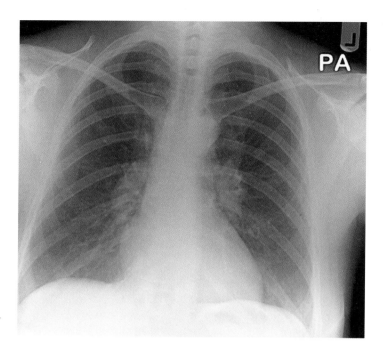

Figure 2.4 Bilateral hilar lymphadenopathy in sarcoidosis.

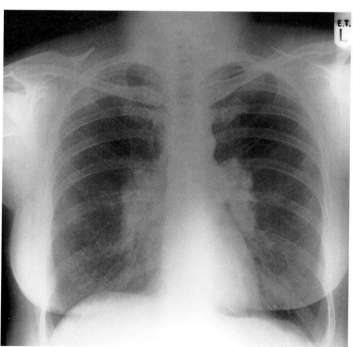

Figure 2.5 A more florid example of bilateral hilar lymphadenopathy, again due to sarcoidosis.

⚡ HAZARD

Note the abnormal shape of the right breast and the metal clips in the right axilla in Fig. 2.3. This woman had undergone surgical treatment for carcinoma of the breast with lumpectomy and axillary lymph node clearance. There are also healing fractures of ribs 3, 4, 5 and 6 on the right, which were fortunately traumatic, not metastatic. Only a systematic approach will ensure that all of these abnormalities are detected.

- If you think the hila may be abnormal, search for additional clues on the radiograph. In Fig. 2.6 paratracheal lymphadenopathy and multiple patches of consolidation can be seen in the lung fields as well as right hilar enlargement – the diagnosis was long-standing sarcoidosis. A mass in the lung fields in addition to an abnormal hilum is highly suggestive of malignancy. Exclude small pleural effusions and look for evidence of a pulmonary infiltrate in association with hilar enlargement (Fig. 2.7).

- These are examples of enlarged hilar shadows but sometimes one or other hilum may appear to be smaller than normal. This is seen (together with hyperlucency of the right lung) in Macleod's syndrome and occasionally in other situations (Fig. 2.8).

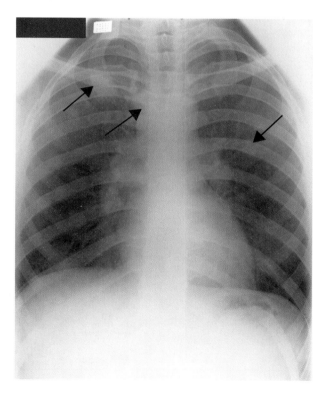

Figure 2.6 Chronic sarcoidosis – paratracheal lymph node enlargement and areas of pulmonary infiltration (both arrowed) in association with bilateral hilar lymphadenopathy.

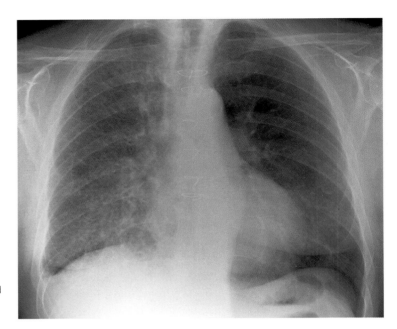

Figure 2.7 The pulmonary infiltrate in the right lung field is due to lymphangitis carcinomatosa and is associated with hilar enlargement and a small pleural effusion. The primary carcinoma was in the breast.

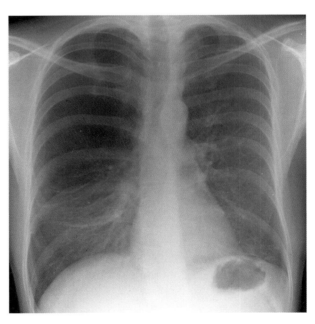

Figure 2.8 An apparently small right hilum, which is pushed downward (the 'y-on-side' is distorted) by a large emphysematous bulla.

PEARL OF WISDOM

Macleod's syndrome: Swyer and James in 1953 and then Macleod, in 1954, described unilateral hyperlucency of one or other lung field and the condition was ascribed to severe neonatal or childhood bronchiolitis, resulting in destruction of lung units during the active period of their development. The chest X-ray is diagnostic with a normal-sized or small lung in association with a small hilum and pulmonary vessels that are distributed sparsely throughout the respective lung field.

CAUSES OF HILAR ENLARGEMENT

Vascular

We have seen illustrations of prominent proximal vascular markings in congenital heart disease and in pulmonary hypertension (the commonest cause of which is chronic obstructive pulmonary disease). Unilateral hilar vascular enlargement can also occur in massive pulmonary embolism when it may be associated with ipsilateral hyperlucency of the lung field (Westermark's sign, see Fig. 6.4, page 131).

Non-vascular

Lymph nodes are usually responsible for non-vascular hilar enlargement and they are commonly accompanied by enlargement of other groups of intrathoracic lymph nodes with a pattern of distribution that can give clues to the pathological diagnosis.

Lymph node enlargement caused by lymphoma and leukaemia

Mediastinal lymph node enlargement is the most common chest radiographic finding in Hodgkin's disease and is seen on the initial chest X-ray of approximately 50 per cent of patients with this condition. In the majority, lymph node involvement is bilateral but asymmetric. Unilateral lymphadenopathy is unusual and paratracheal and subcarinal nodes are involved as often as, or even more commonly than, hilar nodes. Involvement of anterior mediastinal and retrosternal nodes is also common and this anatomic distribution is a major factor in distinguishing lymphoma from sarcoidosis. Sarcoidosis rarely causes radiographically visible nodal enlargement in the anterior mediastinal compartment.

Mediastinal and/or hilar lymph node enlargement is also the commonest intrathoracic manifestation of both non-Hodgkin's lymphoma and leukaemia and, not surprisingly, leukaemic intrathoracic lymphadenopathy is far commoner in the lymphocytic forms of this disease.

Metastatic lymph node enlargement

Lymphomas are responsible for the majority of mediastinal lymph node malignancies but the second most common cause is metastasis from solid tumours, especially from the lungs, upper gastrointestinal tract, prostate, kidneys and genitals.

PEARL OF WISDOM

When the primary lesion is in the lung, mediastinal lymph node enlargement is almost invariably unilateral. Also, the primary lesion may be barely visible or even invisible; this situation is highly suggestive of an oat-cell primary (see Fig. 4.51, page 107).

Lymphadenopathy in granulomatous diseases

Granulomatous conditions include infective causes such as tuberculosis and histoplasmosis (rare in the UK but more common in the USA), as well as sarcoidosis.

In infectious granulomatous diseases, lymphadenopathy tends to be unilateral (Fig. 2.9). There are always exceptions to prove the rule of course and the radiograph in Fig. 2.10 clearly shows bilateral hilar lymphadenopathy in a child with primary tuberculosis.

Although bilateral hilar lymphadenopathy is the norm in sarcoidosis, nodes are often asymmetrically enlarged, with those on the right commonly (though not exclusively) more prominent.

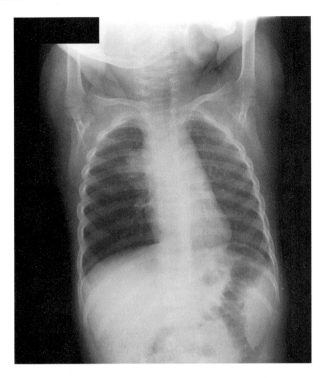

Figure 2.9 Unilateral right hilar and paratracheal lymphadenopathy in a child with primary tuberculosis. The hyperlucency of the right lung field and the mediastinal shift are manifestations of obstructive emphysema, a rare complication of hilar lymph node enlargement caused by extrinsic compression on the right major bronchi.

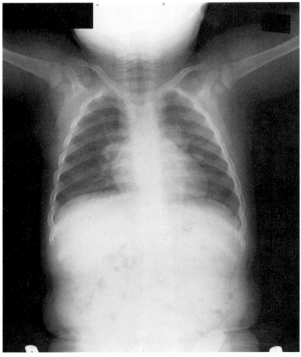

Figure 2.10 Another example of primary tuberculosis in a child. In this case, the hilar nodes are (unusually) symmetrically enlarged.

> ### ● PEARL OF WISDOM
>
> Mediastinal lymph node enlargement in sarcoidosis is almost invariably seen in combination with hilar node involvement and this is an important differentiating feature from lymphoma. Calcification of mediastinal and hilar lymph nodes is highly suggestive of infective or granulomatous aetiology, although the 'egg-shell' pattern of calcification characteristic of sarcoidosis is also seen in silicosis (Figs 2.11 and 2.12).

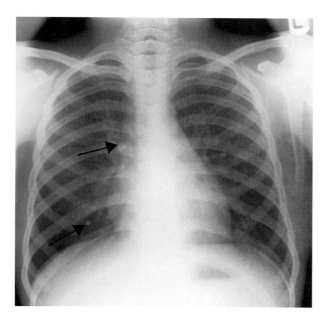

Figure 2.11 Calcified tuberculous complex in a child. At least one Ghon focus can be seen (arrowed) as well as the calcified right hilar lymph nodes.

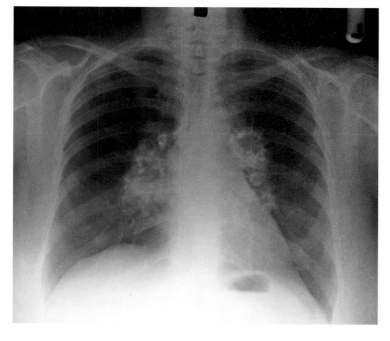

Figure 2.12 Egg-shell calcification in sarcoid lymph nodes.

Unusual causes of mediastinal lymphadenopathy

- Castleman's disease: This condition, also known as angiofollicular hyperplasia was first described by Castleman in 1956. The unicentric variety involves lymph nodes in one geographical area (usually the mediastinum or mesentery). In 90–95 per cent of cases surgical resection is curative and progression to lymphoma or to other tumours is unusual. The multicentric variety carries a worse prognosis and is associated with lymphoma – approximately 50 per cent of cases are caused by caused by Kaposi's sarcoma-associated herpesvirus (KSHV), a gammaherpesvirus that is also the cause of Kaposi's sarcoma.

- Infectious mononucleosis is a rare cause of mediastinal and hilar lymphadenopathy.

MEDIASTINAL GEOGRAPHY

The anatomical boundaries of the mediastinum are the thoracic inlet superiorly, the diaphragm inferiorly and the parietal pleura (investing the medial surfaces of the lungs) on both sides laterally.

Figure 2.13 is a diagrammatic representation, shown in left lateral view, of three hypothetical mediastinal areas and the organs they contain. Dividing the mediastinum into compartments in this way, together with a consideration of the anatomical structures contained within each, assists in the differential diagnosis of abnormal mediastinal shadowing. Table 2.1 extends this anatomical approach and lists mediastinal masses according to compartment.

Table 2.1 Mediastinal masses, tabulated according to compartment (see text)

Anterior compartment	Middle compartment	Posterior compartment	More than one compartment
Retrosternal thyroid	Pericardial cyst	Neural tumour	Lymphoma
Thymic masses	Aortic aneurysm	Oesophagus	Metastatic solid
• hyperplasia	Anomalous or	• tumour	tumour
• cyst	ectatic vessels	• achalasia	Sarcoidosis
• thymoma	Left ventricular	• gastroenteric cyst	Tuberculosis
Germ cell tumours	aneurysm	Trachea	Castleman's disease
• benign (dermoid)	Cardiomegaly	• bronchogenic cyst	Bronchial and
• malignant		Hiatus hernia	gastroenteric cysts
Lymphoma		Bochdalek hernia	
Other malignancies		Descending aorta	
Morgagni hernia		aneurysm	

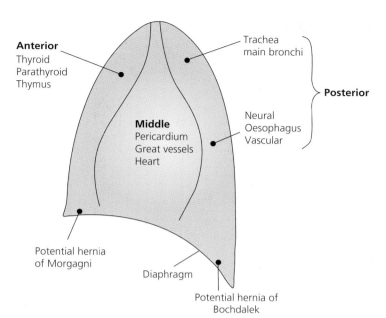

Figure 2.13 Diagram of the mediastinum shown in left lateral view, showing the organs residing in the anterior, middle and posterior compartments, respectively.

- The anterior compartment is bounded by the sternum anteriorly, the pericardium posteriorly and the diaphragm inferiorly.
- The anterior boundary of the posterior compartment is the posterior surface of the pericardium. Posteriorly it abuts on the vertebral bodies and the paravertebral gutters and, inferiorly, it reaches the diaphragm.
- The middle compartment is bounded by the pericardium.
- The three compartments come together and become less well defined in the superior mediastinum.

Examples of mediastinal masses

Figure 2.14 shows a large retrosternal thyroid goitre with concentric narrowing of the trachea. The extent of the extrinsic tracheal compression is shown dramatically in Fig. 2.15, which is a CT scan of the same patient.

Figures 2.16 and 2.17 are the chest radiograph and CT scan, respectively, of a young man with Hodgkin's lymphoma. Comparing this radiograph with Fig. 2.14, one can see a more defined upper border whereas the thyroid mass continues up to and merges with the thoracic inlet.

The bronchogenic cyst illustrated in Figs 2.18 and 2.19 has a different shape again. In all fairness, one could not reliably differentiate this from lymphoma on the chest X-ray alone but the more posterior position of the mass on CT scan is more reassuring of its benign nature.

The anterior mediastinal mass clearly shown in Figs 2.20 and 2.21 developed in a middle-aged woman who had myasthenia gravis. Not surprisingly, this proved to be a thymoma.

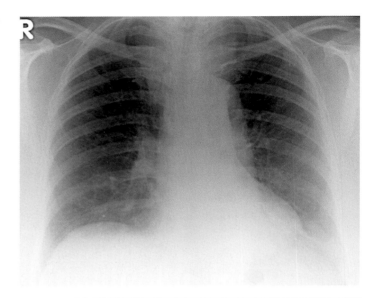

Figure 2.14 Retrosternal thyroid goitre surrounding and compressing the trachea.

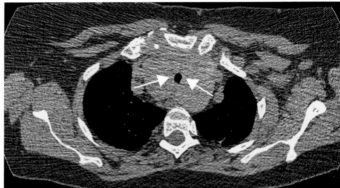

Figure 2.15 CT scan of the patient in Fig. 2.14, showing marked, concentric narrowing of the trachea.

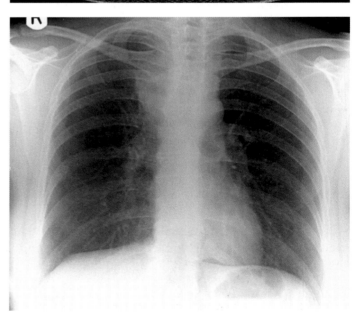

Figure 2.16 Hodgkin's lymphoma with a right paratracheal mass of lymph nodes.

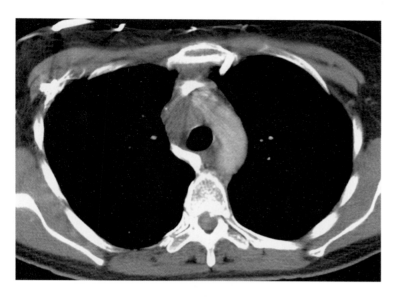

Figure 2.17 CT scan of the patient shown in Fig. 2.16.

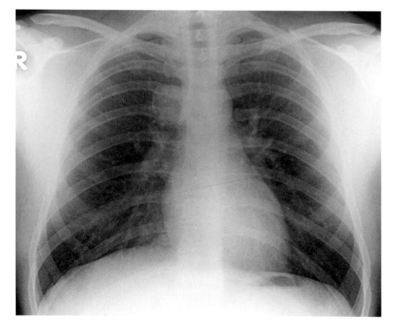

Figure 2.18 Bronchogenic cyst.

PEARL OF WISDOM

The thymus is an anterior mediastinal structure but thymomas often extend up into the superior mediastinum. Indeed, they may appear as predominantly superior mediastinal masses.

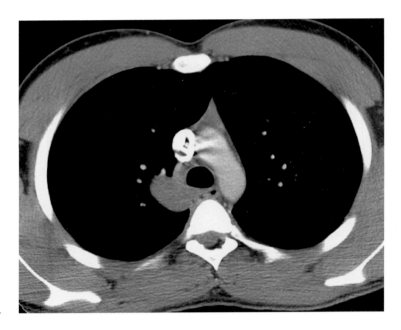

Figure 2.19 CT scan of the bronchogenic cyst shown in Fig. 2.18.

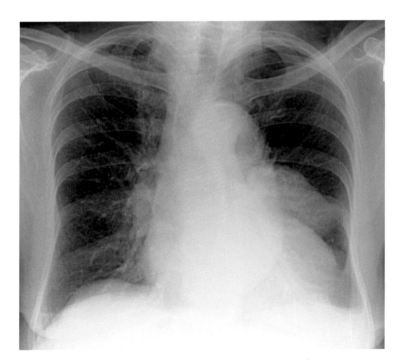

Figure 2.20 Thymoma in a patient with myasthenia gravis.

The young man whose chest X-ray is the subject of Fig. 2.22 presented on our acute medical 'take' with chest pain. The radiograph was fairly unimpressive but suspicions were raised by the rather obscure left heart border (a tribute to the systematic approach) and the subsequent CT scan (Fig. 2.23) was highly abnormal, showing a large anterior mediastinal mass. This turned out to be a malignant teratoma.

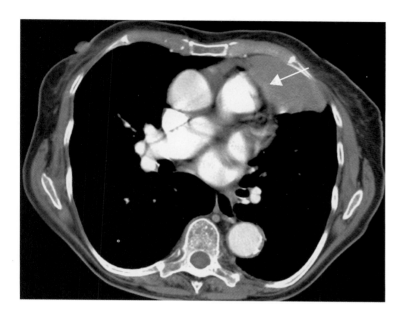

Figure 2.21 CT scan of the patient shown in Fig. 2.20, showing the large anterior mediastinal mass (arrowed).

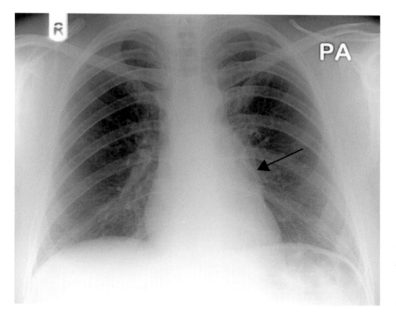

Figure 2.22 Teratoma creating an anterior mediastinal mass. The subtle lack of definition of the left heart border is the clue to a mediastinal abnormality here.

Figure 2.24 is an obviously abnormal chest X-ray and the clinical diagnosis was not difficult as this 55-year-old man presented with central chest pain radiating to his back. The aortic dissection was confirmed on the CT scan depicted in Fig. 2.25 and the patient made an excellent recovery with surgery.

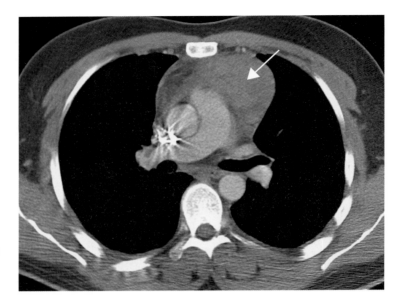

Figure 2.23 The subsequent CT scan of the patient shown in Fig. 2.22 was highly abnormal (the teratoma is arrowed).

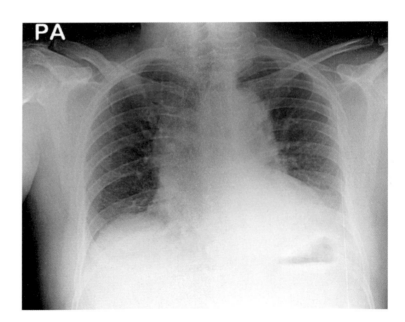

Figure 2.24 Aortic dissection with a widened mediastinum.

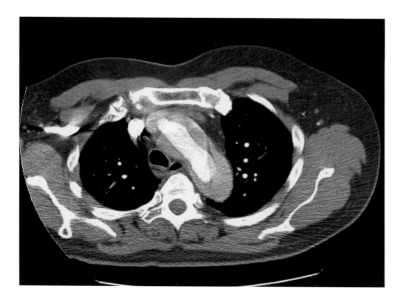

Figure 2.25 CT scan of the patient shown in Fig. 2.24.

⚡ HAZARD

The chest X-ray is commonly normal in aortic dissection and it is essential to maintain a high index of suspicion of this diagnosis. Chest pain that radiates to the back should always raise the possibility of dissection and remember that a dissection can track proximally as well as distally to involve the carotid arteries (associated pain in the neck) and even the coronary ostia, resulting in primary cardiac pain and even myocardial infarction. Any suspicion should flag the need for mediastinal CT imaging.

Identifying posterior mediastinal masses can be difficult, particularly if the shadowing is behind the heart. See Figs 1.27 and 1.28 (pages 19 and 20) as an example.

Check List Chapter 2

✓ Examine the hilar shadows. Identify the mid-point of each hilum and measure its diameter. Remember the landmarks for normal hilar position on each side and decide if there is shift upwards or downwards, suggesting loss of volume in the respective lobe of lung.

✓ The hila resemble the letter 'y' on its side. Examine them for any distortion of this shape.

✓ If you suspect hilar enlargement, attempt to decide if this is vascular or non-vascular and look for additional abnormalities in the lung fields and pleura.

✓ Have a high index of suspicion of abnormality in the mediastinum; changes on chest X-ray can be very subtle and further imaging may be necessary.

✓ Consider the mediastinum in separate geographic departments and learn the anatomical components of each. This assists the differential diagnosis of masses originating in each area.

✓ The chest X-ray is a fairly coarse tool in identifying hilar and mediastinal pathology and it is vital to consider a patient's clinical presentation along with the radiographic appearances when determining the need for further investigation.

CHAPTER 3

Consolidation, collapse and cavitation

This chapter discusses the radiographic patterns of pulmonary consolidation and illustrates the various pathological processes that can cause it. It also describes the features of partial and complete collapse of the major lobes of the lungs. We are all aware that it may be difficult to decide if there is abnormal parenchymal shadowing on a chest radiograph and most of us will also have missed subtle changes of lobar collapse at some stage in our careers. However, there is a systematic approach to the identification of both consolidation and collapse, and in this chapter I seek to share it. I guarantee that if the system is adopted and practised then eventually 'pattern recognition' will take over – in other words, 'I have seen this pattern of abnormality lots of times before and I know what it is'. However, before any of us reaches this stage of experience, it is vital to be obsessional about following a systematic approach – but then this applies to all aspects of clinical medicine.

DEFINITIONS

Consolidation

Consolidation is a pathological term. It describes the state of the lung when alveolar gas has been replaced by fluid, cells or a mixture of the two. Various terms have been used in an attempt to describe the morphological appearance of consolidation – 'alveolar-filling pattern', 'air-space filling' and 'ground-glass shadowing' are examples. I prefer the first of these because it is so descriptive and I use it preferentially in this chapter.

Whatever the terminology, the radiographic appearances of consolidation are those of homogeneous shadowing in part of the lung field with little or no lobar shrinkage. The normal vascular pattern is lost because the alveolar-filling process denies the definition of lung markings by replacing the air in adjacent lung parenchyma. This loss of vascular pattern is a major clue when the appearances of consolidation are subtle.

It is important to remember that none of these terms can determine the pathological nature of the substance that has resulted in the appearance of alveolar filling. An identical radiographic pattern can be the result of bacterial infection, the transudate of heart failure, alveolar haemorrhage, pneumonia due to *Pneumocystis carinii* or the malignant infiltrate of alveolar cell carcinoma. However, there are additional clues on a radiograph that can narrow the pathological diagnosis and one should seek these out. An example is the classical distribution of consolidation in chronic eosinophilic pneumonia. Described as 'reverse pulmonary oedema', the radiographic appearance is virtually diagnostic with predominantly peripheral consolidation that crosses boundaries between individual lobes and segments (Fig. 3.1).

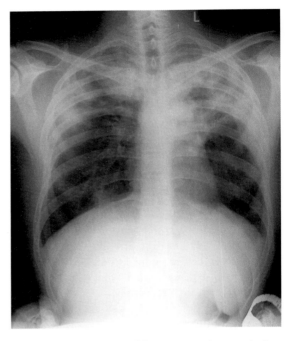

Figure 3.1 An example of eosinophilic pneumonia.

Another example, discussed in the Preface, is an alveolar-filling pattern in association with pleural effusions, cardiomegaly and interstitial lines – a combination that virtually secures the diagnosis of heart failure (Figs 1 and 2, page viii).

CLINICAL CONNECTIONS

Heart failure is usually associated with cardiomegaly, but not exclusively so. Normal heart size may be retained in the following circumstances:

- if heart failure is of sudden onset, a classic example being mitral valve rupture after myocardial infarction
- restrictive cardiomyopathy
- pericardial constriction
- mitral valve disease – when rheumatic heart disease was prevalent, mitral stenosis regularly progressed to cause left atrial failure, the X-ray manifestations of which are identical to left ventricular failure.

Collapse

Consolidated lung may lose volume at any stage in disease progression but the crucial question is whether consolidation is secondary to collapse. The obvious cause of this is major airway obstruction and this has important management implications. Marked loss of volume on the radiograph is likely to indicate pathology causing primary collapse and should be investigated as such.

When the primary process is consolidation, on the other hand, any subsequent loss of volume is not usually dramatic unless the disease is a chronic infective one such as tuberculosis or chronic *Klebsiella* pneumonia. One of the reasons for emphasizing this point is to question the value of the compromise term 'consolidation collapse'. To use this description seems scarcely worthwhile because it does not assist in deciding whether bronchial occlusion is present and therefore fails to materially guide patient management.

Density

When referring to radiographic shadowing, the term 'density' refers to the radio-opacity of a lesion and this will be influenced fundamentally by the degree of exposure of the film. With this important qualification and assuming ideal radiographic exposure of the image, I think it is useful to consider three grades of density as follows:

- **low density** – small shadows caused by cells or body fluids
- **medium density** – larger shadows especially caused by fluids
- **high density** – shadows containing radio-opaque atoms either derived from body fluids (iron or calcium) or introduced from the environment (iron, calcium, barium or tin).

Inevitably, these distinctions will be subjective to a certain extent and, in particular, the separation of low- and medium-density shadows can be difficult but the classification is still helpful and I would recommend it to you.

A SYSTEMATIC APPROACH TO CONSOLIDATION (OR ALVEOLAR FILLING)

Ensure that the abnormal shadowing represents an alveolar-filling process

Extensive pulmonary infiltrates of various types can coalesce and mimic 'alveolar filling'. Examine the nature of the shadowing carefully – is it truly homogeneous or does it appear to be a coalescence of rounded shadows (nodular), streaky shadows (reticular) or a combination of the two (reticulo-nodular)? The intrapulmonary shadowing in Fig. 3.2 is certainly generalized and may appear homogeneous at first

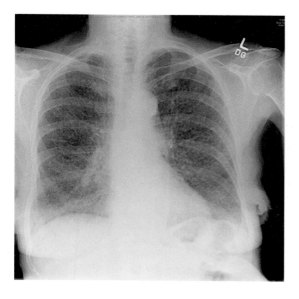

Figure 3.2 Miliary tuberculosis.

sight but closer inspection reveals that it is made up of myriads of tiny dots in all areas of the lung fields. It almost looks as though someone has scattered the contents of a salt-cellar over the film – this is an example of military tuberculosis.

What is the distribution of the abnormal shadowing?

Lobar pneumonia affects lobes or segments uniformly (Figs 3.3 and 3.4). Although pneumonia caused by a variety of infecting agents, including *Pneumococcus*, can

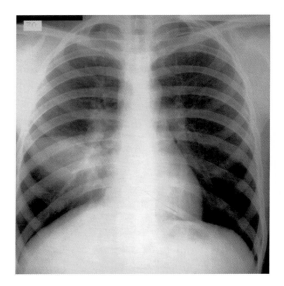

Figure 3.3 Pneumococcal pneumonia affecting the right middle lobe. The consolidation has a sharp upper border where it abuts the horizontal fissure. The heart border is lost, indicating that this is anterior shadowing and therefore confirming middle lobe involvement. There is no air bronchogram, which can happen with pneumococcal and other bacterial pneumonias (staphylococcal and Gram-negatives especially) when exudate fills the airways as well as the lung parenchyma.

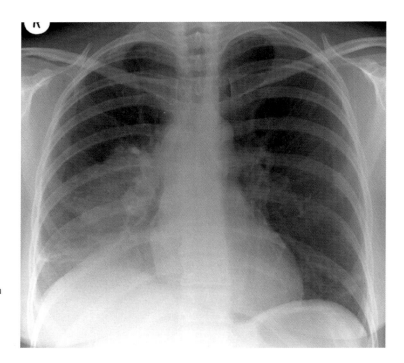

Figure 3.4 Pneumococcal pneumonia in the right lower lobe. This time the heart border is preserved, the upper boundary is indistinct and the right hemidiaphragm is blurred.

affect multiple lobes or segments, the radiographic appearance of multiple segmental or subsegmental consolidation should arouse diagnostic suspicion of non-infective aetiology:

- If the shadowing is predominantly peripheral, eosinophilic pneumonia should be considered (Fig. 3.5). In the majority of cases, a circulating eosinophilia provides a clue to the diagnosis but this isn't always present and lung biopsy may be needed to confirm the nature of the eosinophilic infiltrate.
- Other non-infective but inflammatory conditions cause multisegmental consolidation. Figure 3.6 is an example of cryptogenic organizing pneumonitis, an inflammatory condition with a clinical presentation that commonly mimics pneumonia.
- Both of these conditions require treatment with corticosteroids, emphasizing the management implications of distinguishing non-infective causes of consolidation.
- Wegener's granulomatosis is a vasculitic disease, which characteristically produces multiple areas of consolidation when it affects the lungs. These lesions commonly cavitate (Fig. 3.7).
- On rare occasions, sarcoidosis causes multisegmental consolidation (Fig. 3.8). In Fig. 3.9 there are nodules as well as patches of consolidation.
- Malignant infiltrates (haematological, lymphoproliferative and solid tissue tumours) are also in the differential diagnosis of multisegmental consolidation.

⚡ HAZARD

Consider non-infective pathology if there are multiple areas of consolidation. A thorough interpretation of the radiograph will raise your suspicions and help to ensure early appropriate treatment. Even though the story may sound like infection, this radiographic pattern can also be caused by disease processes that will not respond to antibiotics.

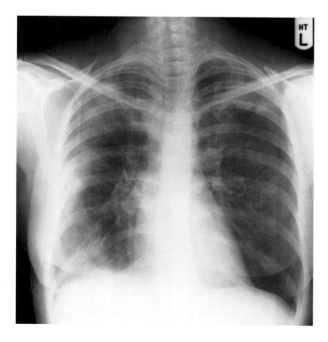

Figure 3.5 Eosinophilic pneumonia. The peripheral consolidation in this example is asymmetric with involvement of all areas of the right lung but only the apex on the left.

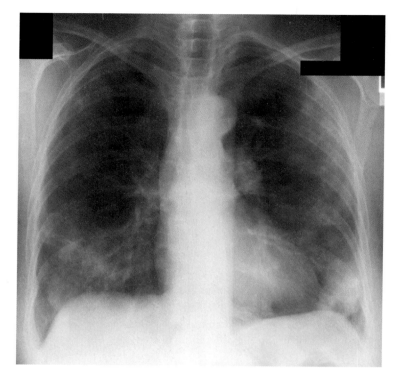

Figure 3.6 Cryptogenic organizing pneumonitis. Suspicion regarding the original diagnosis of pneumonia arose when no organism was identified and there was a lack of response to antibiotics. The correct diagnosis was made on lung biopsy.

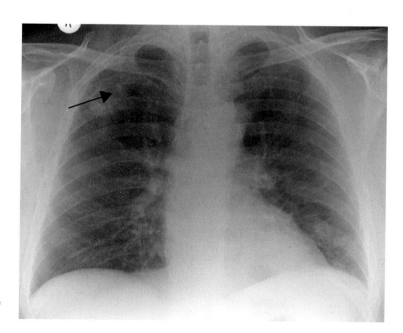

Figure 3.7 Wegener's granulomatosis. There are patches of consolidation in the right upper and left lower zones and cavitation can be seen in the former.

3 Consolidation, collapse and cavitation

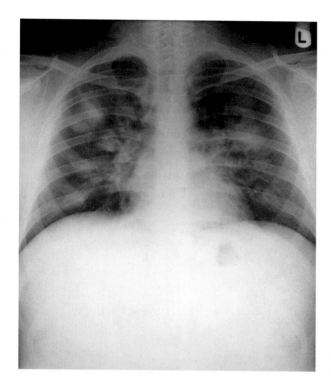

Figure 3.8 Bilateral multiple segmental consolidation in sarcoidosis.

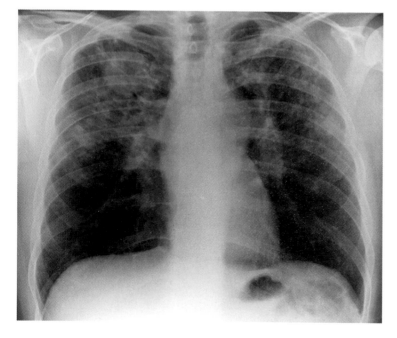

Figure 3.9 Nodules are present as well as confluent areas of consolidation. The bilateral hilar lymphadenopathy is a clue to the diagnosis of sarcoidosis.

Other recognizable radiographic patterns include:

- Pulmonary oedema. This has a characteristic perihilar distribution and the epithet, 'Bat's wing of death', though unfortunate, is often appropriate morphologically (Fig. 3.10).

- Aspiration pneumonia is one cause of bilateral consolidation in the lower zones. Loss of volume may accompany the consolidation as a result of bronchial obstruction from aspirated.

- Alveolar haemorrhage is commonly perihilar in distribution but this isn't totally reliable – the major haemorrhage shown in Fig. 3.11 has resulted in extensive

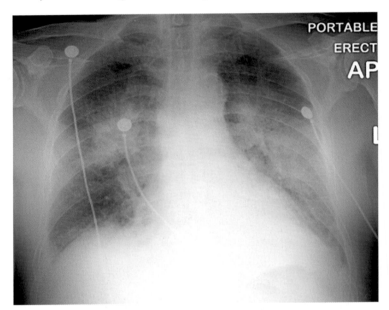

Figure 3.10 Pulmonary oedema – the 'bat's-wing' appearance.

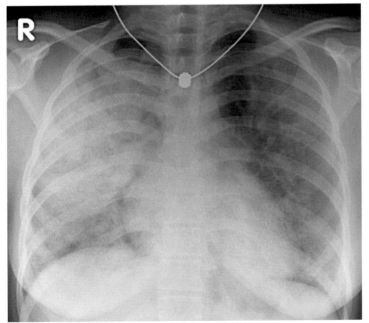

Figure 3.11 Extensive intrapulmonary haemorrhage in a patient with idiopathic pulmonary haemosiderosis.

bilateral consolidation. There is no air-bronchogram within the shadowing because blood is filling the airways as well as the alveoli.

In contrast:

- There are no distinguishing radiographic features displayed by the bilateral alveolar filling pattern in the example of pulmonary alveolar proteinosis shown in Fig. 3.12 and the same applies to most cases of *Pneumocystis carinii* pneumonia (Fig. 3.13) and alveolar cell carcinoma (Fig. 3.14). The consolidation in Fig. 3.15 is as a result of the adult respiratory distress syndrome and, although the multitude of tubes and wires may be a clue as to aetiology, there is nothing diagnostic about the radiograph per se.

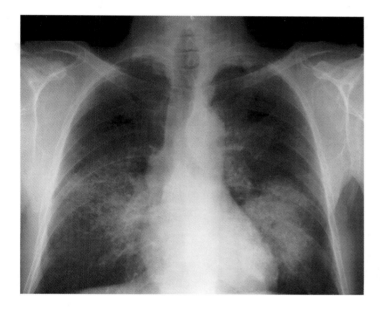

Figure 3.12 Pulmonary alveolar proteinosis.

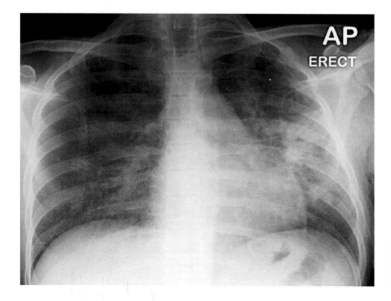

Figure 3.13 Extensive bilateral alveolar-filling pattern in *Pneumocystis carinii* pneumonia complicating human immunodeficiency virus (HIV) infection.

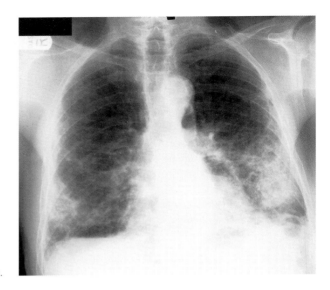

Figure 3.14 Alveolar cell carcinoma.

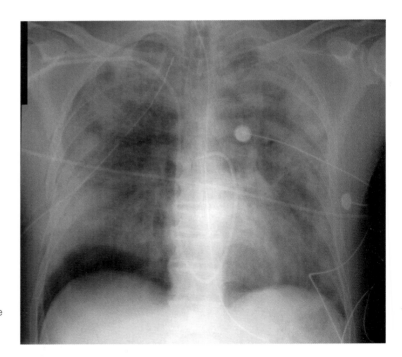

Figure 3.15 Adult respiratory distress syndrome. The pulmonary flotation catheter, nasogastric and endotracheal tubes, intercostal chest drain and electrocardiogram wires are a give-away that this film was taken on an intensive care unit.

CLINICAL CONNECTIONS

The last four cases illustrate the fact that lungs become consolidated in a variety of pathological conditions and that the radiographic appearance of 'alveolar filling' is ubiquitous and non-discriminatory in many instances.

What is the density of the shadowing?

Sometimes consolidation is of low density, but more commonly it is medium dense, representing as it does alveoli filled with fluid, cells, infective organisms or a mixture of these components. Heavy-density shadowing is not seen except under unusual circumstances, for example if a radiodense foreign body is responsible for bronchial obstruction (see Clinical connections).

CLINICAL CONNECTIONS

A middle-aged man with a heavy alcohol intake presented one weekend septic with pneumonia. He had consolidation with no air bronchogram in the right middle and lower lobes and there appeared to be a calcified area approximately 1 cm² in the right mid-zone. At bronchoscopy, I retrieved a vertebral body of a small mammal (presumably a rabbit) from the intermediate bronchus. He recovered remarkably well despite the fact that *Actinomyces* was present in bronchial aspirate. Although he had no recollection of eating rabbit or anything similar, this was presumably aspiration pneumonia.

Cavitation within an area of consolidation indicates a particular infecting organism (*Staphylococcus*, *Mycobacteria* and Gram-negative organisms are in the differential diagnosis [Figs 3.16 and 3.17], bronchial obstruction with distal cavitation complicating a bronchial carcinoma [Fig. 3.18] or foreign body) or a completely different pathologic process, for example primary lung abscess (Fig. 3.19) or a cavitating pulmonary infarct.

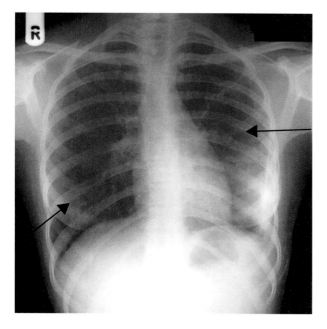

Figure 3.16 Staphylococcal septicaemia with multiple areas of consolidation, several of which are starting to cavitate (arrowed).

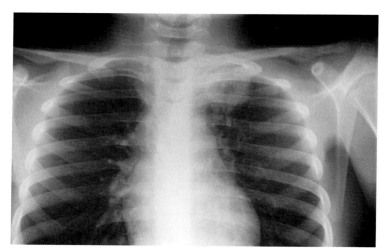

Figure 3.17 Tuberculosis. A left cavity is clearly seen in the apical consolidation.

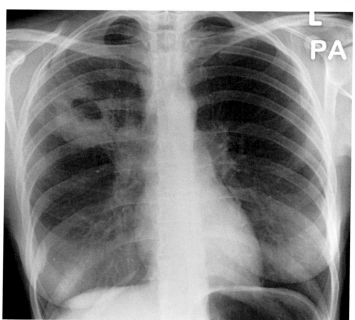

Figure 3.18 Cavitating squamous cell carcinoma.

Is there an associated 'air bronchogram'?

An air bronchogram is created by the persistence of air-filled bronchi travelling through an area of consolidated lung, looking like the branches of a tree after autumn's leaf fall. Figure 3.20 is an example.

CLINICAL CONNECTIONS

The presence or absence of an air bronchogram provides clues as to the underlying pathology. When absent, it indicates that the airways have become filled with material of equivalent radiodensity to that of the surrounding consolidated lung. Absence of an air bronchogram in association with extensive consolidation suggests either an infective process with large amounts of secretions (the classic examples being pneumococcal (see Fig. 3.3, page 48) or staphylococcal pneumonia) or consolidation in association with proximal bronchial obstruction (carcinoma, foreign body, aspiration and so on, Figs 3.21 and 3.22).

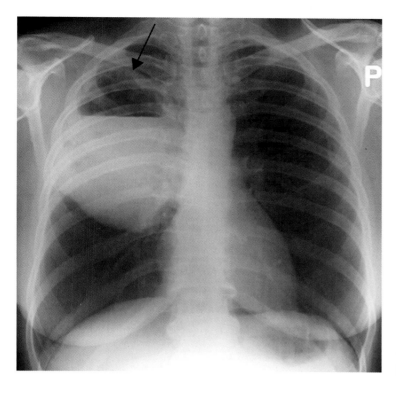

Figure 3.19 Primary lung abscess; note the thick upper wall (arrowed).

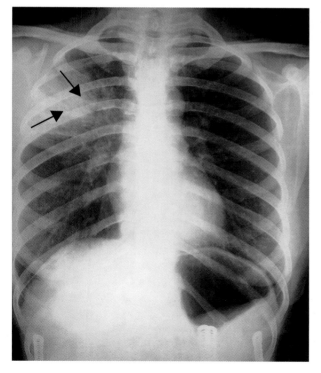

Figure 3.20 The air bronchogram is arrowed in this case of pneumococcal pneumonia affecting the posterior segment of the right upper lobe.

3 Consolidation, collapse and cavitation

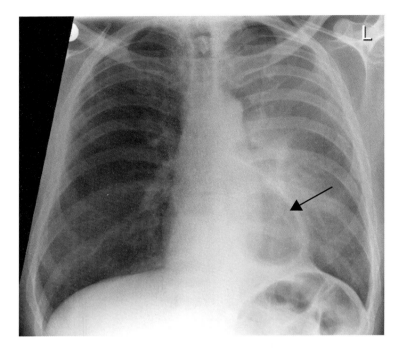

Figure 3.21 Left upper lobe consolidation (and a minor degree of collapse). There is no air bronchogram. Note the large hiatus hernia (arrowed) – this was aspiration pneumonia with obstruction of the left upper lobe bronchus by gastric contents.

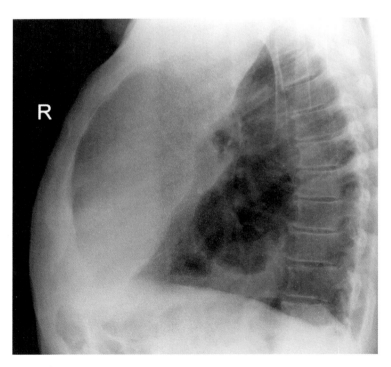

Figure 3.22 Lateral view of Fig. 3.21.

Is there radiographic evidence of other disease?

Look for lymphadenopathy, bony abnormalities (Fig. 3.23) and pleural shadowing.

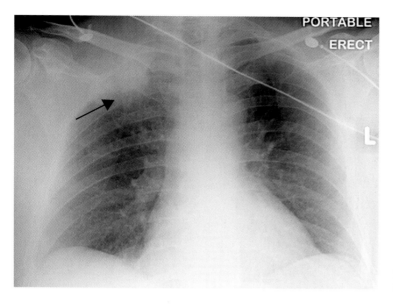

Figure 3.23 Pancoast tumour destroying first and second rib.

> ### CLINICAL CONNECTIONS
>
> A unilateral pleural effusion in the presence of consolidation may suggest underlying malignancy or, alternatively, indicate empyema formation. Both of these possibilities demand early investigation with further imaging (ultrasound scan and/or computed tomography [CT] scan) and diagnostic pleural aspiration with or without pleural biopsy.

Is consolidation accompanied by significant collapse?

Marked loss of volume of consolidated lung is highly suggestive of underlying, often malignant, disease and also rings alarm bells for further investigation. With this in mind, a logical next step is to consider a systematic diagnostic approach to pulmonary collapse.

COLLAPSE

An important part of this exercise is to look at examples of collapse of all the major lobes, examine them repeatedly and start to develop skills of 'pattern recognition'. In addition to this, though, there are a few basic points to consider:

- If a lobe collapses completely, it may become radiographically invisible. Figure 3.24 is an example; an occluding bronchial carcinoma has resulted in total collapse of the right upper lobe, which has virtually disappeared. Under these circumstances, one has to rely on the ancillary radiographic changes of 'loss of normal lines and shadows' and 'shift of normal structures' to make the diagnosis. These are discussed below.

- On the other hand, complete collapse of the left lower lobe almost invariably leaves a characteristic line behind the heart and this appearance should stimulate you to search for confirmatory radiographic signs of loss of volume in this lobe (Fig. 3.25).

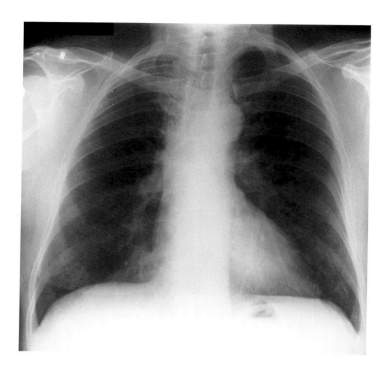

Figure 3.24 Complete collapse of right upper lobe.

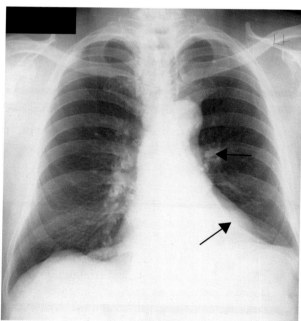

Figure 3.25 Left lower lobe collapse. The characteristic line behind the heart is arrowed and note also the calcified hilar lymph nodes of old tuberculosis. The glands on the left clearly indicate that the hilum is pulled downwards on this side, supporting the diagnosis of left lower lobe collapse.

- A lateral chest X-ray may help to confirm major collapse, particularly of middle lobe and lingula (see Figs 3.34 and 3.36, pages 66 and 67, respectively) but in other instances it can be disappointingly unhelpful and this applies especially to the lower lobes (Fig. 3.26).

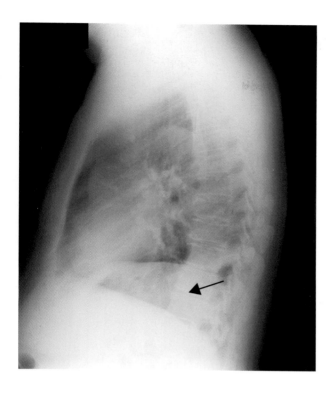

Figure 3.26 Left lateral view of Fig. 3.25. The clues to left lower lobe pathology are the elevated left hemidiaphragm and the shadow superimposed on vertebral bodies (arrowed) – this is produced by the solid left lower lobe.

The radiographic signs of collapse

There are three categories of radiographic signs that contribute to the recognition of lobar collapse:

1. The shadow created by the abnormal lobe itself. As we have seen this may be of little help if the offending lobe has collapsed completely.

2. Loss of normal lines and shadows. The lines created by anatomical structures will become blurred if abnormal, non-aerated lung collapses against them. For example, the medial part of the respective hemidiaphragm becomes indistinct in the presence of collapse of one or other lower lobe (see Figs 3.37 and 3.38, page 68). Similarly, there is loss (or blurring) of the respective heart border in middle lobe consolidation (see Fig. 3.32, page 65), collapse (see Fig. 3.33, page 65) and lingular collapse (see Figs 3.35, pages 67), the paravertebral structures become indistinct in lower lobe collapse (see Figs 3.37 and 3.38, page 68) and so does the right upper mediastinum in right upper lobe collapse as illustrated in Fig. 3.24.

3. Shift of normal structures. The hilum is pulled downwards by collapse of the ipsilateral lower lobe and upwards by loss of volume in the upper lobe.

> ### PEARL OF WISDOM
>
> Examples of 'shift of normal structures'
> - When the middle lobe loses volume, the horizontal fissure and the right oblique fissure move together but the former tends to move more (see Fig. 3.33, page 65). The hilum may therefore be pulled slightly downwards. However, if the downward movement is more marked, one should be suspicious of combined right middle and right lower lobe collapse, a picture that strongly suggests obstruction of the intermediate bronchus.
> - One or other hemidiaphragm may move upward in association with lobar collapse (see Figs 3.31 and 3.38, pages 64 and 68, respectively).
> - Mediastinal structures can shift to the side of major loss of volume, particularly with complete lung collapse (Fig. 3.27). The tracheal shift towards the abnormal side is clearly illustrated in Fig. 3.27 and is crucial in distinguishing collapsed lung from massive pleural effusion (see Chapter 5).

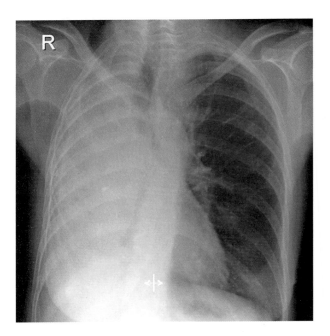

Figure 3.27 Carcinoma of the right main bronchus resulting in complete collapse of the right lung. The mediastinal shift is obvious and the trachea is deviated markedly to the abnormal side.

Examples of lobar collapse

Right upper lobe

Complete collapse (see Fig. 3.24, page 60) results in blurring of the right upper mediastinal shadows and upward shift of the right hilum. The lobe itself virtually disappears. In comparison, the characteristic shadow caused by partial collapse of the right upper lobe as it moves anteriorly and medially is shown in Fig. 3.28.

Left upper lobe

The left upper lobe creates an unmistakeable pattern as it loses volume (shown in Fig. 3.29) and it rarely disappears completely. Note from Fig. 3.29 that the consolidated lobe becomes progressively less dense from top to bottom. This is simply a reflection

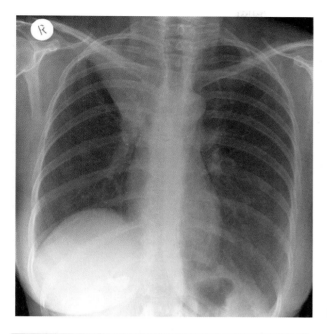

Figure 3.28 Partial collapse of the right upper lobe.

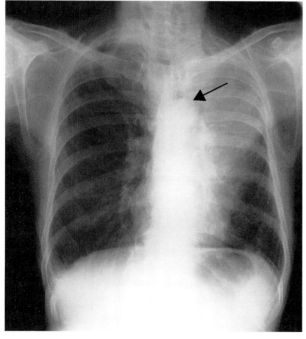

Figure 3.29 Left upper lobe collapse.

of the depth of lung tissue contained within it at different levels. Figure 3.30 is the lateral view of Fig. 3.29, illustrating the predominantly anterior movement of the left oblique fissure. The consolidated lobe shown in Fig. 3.31 has not collapsed to the same extent and the abnormal shadowing extends further down the left hemithorax as a result. Note the hallmark 'comma' of aerated lung outlining the aortic knuckle (arrowed in Figs 3.29 and 3.31). This is probably derived from normal left lung herniating across the mid-line – an example of 'shift of normal structures'. The

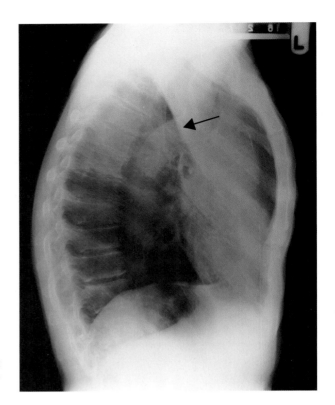

Figure 3.30 Lateral view of Fig. 3.29; the oblique fissure is arrowed. (Note that this lateral film is pictured the wrong way around – a left lateral chest X-ray should be viewed as if looking at the patient's left side and opposite for a right lateral film.)

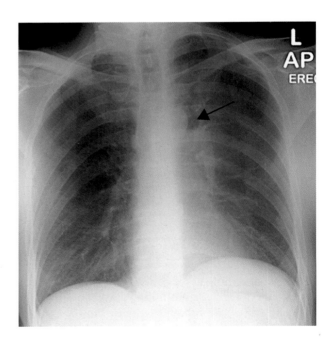

Figure 3.31 Left upper lobe collapse with upward shift of the left hemidiaphragm. The 'comma' of aerated lung around the aortic knuckle, as mentioned in the text, is arrowed.

large hiatus hernia may have been connected with the lung abnormalities because aspirated stomach contents were found at bronchoscopy.

Middle lobe

Figure 3.32 is an example of right middle lobe consolidation with minimal loss of volume. In contrast, the near total right middle lobe collapse depicted in Fig. 3.33

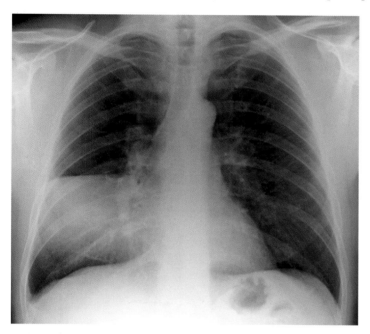

Figure 3.32 Right middle lobe consolidation.

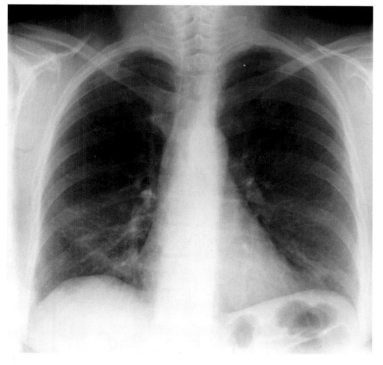

Figure 3.33 Near total collapse of right middle lobe with a patch of shadowing adjacent to the heart border. The clue is the lack of definition of the heart border.

has resulted in minimal abnormality on chest X-ray in posterio-anterior (PA) view, with just a small area of shadowing adjacent to the right border, which is partially obliterated. The right lateral X-ray of the same patient (Fig. 3.34) is strikingly abnormal, emphasizing the need to have a high index of suspicion of middle lobe pathology on PA chest radiograph.

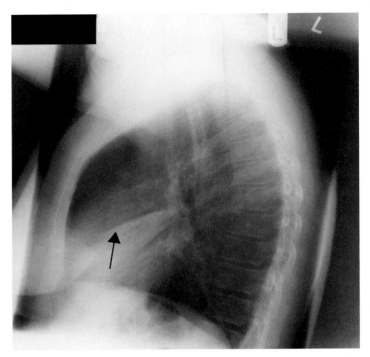

Figure 3.34 Lateral radiograph of the patient shown in Fig. 3.33. The collapsed middle lobe is arrowed and note that the horizontal fissure has moved downward and the oblique fissure upward.

Lingula

A high index of suspicion is equally necessary when identifying lingular collapse. This is illustrated in Figs 3.35 and 3.36 where the discrepancy between the abnormality seen on PA view compared with that on lateral view is even more striking.

Right lower lobe

Figure 3.37 is an example of complete collapse of the right lower lobe. The characteristic 'sail-shape' shadow can be seen and the right hilum is shifted downward. In addition, the right paravertebral structures and the right hemidiaphragm are both obscured by the abnormally solid right lower lobe that is adjacent to them.

Left lower lobe

Figure 3.38 is an example of left lower lobe collapse and illustrates the three cardinal signs of collapse, the line behind the heart due to the collapsed lobe itself (arrowed), downward displacement of the left hilum ('shift of normal structures') and loss of definition of both left hemidiaphragm and left paravertebral area ('loss of normal lines and shadows').

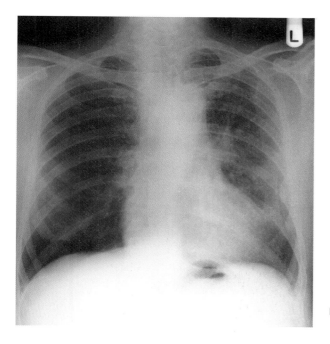

Figure 3.35 Lingular collapse, PA view.

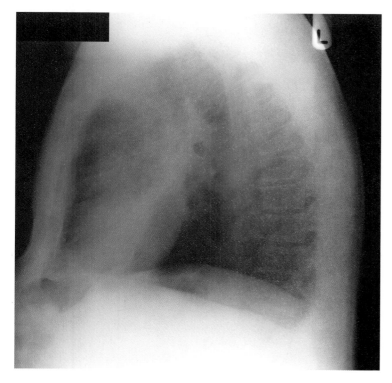

Figure 3.36 Lingular collapse, lateral view.

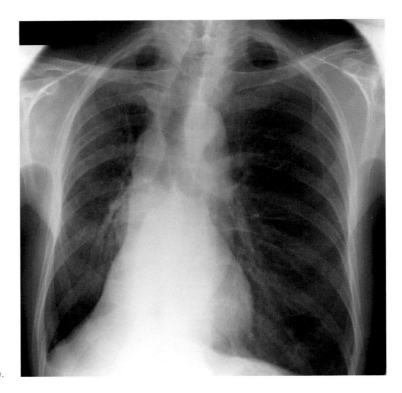

Figure 3.37 Right lower lobe collapse.

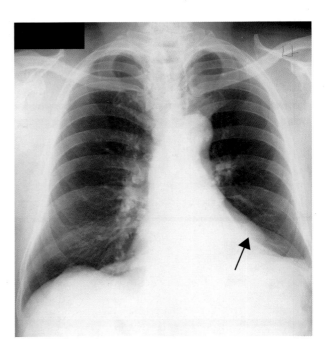

Figure 3.38 Left lower lobe collapse. The line behind the heart that represents the abnormal lobe is arrowed.

CAVITATION

The radiographic appearance of cavitation is created by destruction of tissue within existing abnormal areas of lung and it follows that cavities usually have thick-walled boundaries. This serves to distinguish them from conditions causing thin-walled ring shadows and these are covered in the next chapter.

Many different pathologic processes in the lung can result in cavitation and we have seen a number of examples already (see Figs 3.16–3.19, pages 55–57).

> **CLINICAL CONNECTIONS**
>
> Some bacteria are particularly prone to cause cavitating pneumonia: *Staphylococcus*, mycobacteria, Gram-negative organisms and occasionally the pneumococcus.

A discussion of some of the pathological causes of cavitation follows with notes on the particular radiographic features of each.

Tuberculosis

Post-primary infection is the variety of tuberculosis that typically cavitates although, occasionally, primary foci of infection can progress in this way (see Fig. 3.17, page 56). Post-primary disease tends to affect the apical and posterior parts of the lungs with potential involvement in this distribution in both upper and lower lobes.

> **PEARL OF WISDOM**
>
> This anatomical distribution is explained by the ventilation–perfusion relationship of different parts of the lungs. Mycobacteria like to be ventilated but not perfused – conditions pertaining in the apical regions of each major lobe. This preference is further illustrated in bats, animals that spend a large part of their life hanging upside down – they have foci of mycobacterial infection at their lung bases! It also explains why various surgical treatments for tuberculosis were successful in the pre-antibiotic era, surgical treatments for tuberculosis were successful (artificial pneumothorax, thoracoplasty and plombage (e.g. see Fig. 7.12, page 143). They were all based on the principle of 'resting' infected areas of lung thereby reducing the degree of ventilation within them.

Post-primary tuberculosis usually causes considerable lung fibrosis, as well as caseating necrosis, and these factors conspire to produce a radiographic picture that is typical with bilateral upper zone fibrosis, shrinkage and cavitation (Fig. 3.39). However, other conditions can mimic these appearances and they are discussed in Chapter 4.

Aspergilloma

The fungus ball of *Aspergillus*, also known as a mycetoma, is an opportunist development. The fungus traditionally grows in old tuberculous cavities but can in fact colonize any area of devitalized lung – there are well-documented examples in cavities caused by chronic sarcoidosis and in those associated with ankylosing spondylitis.

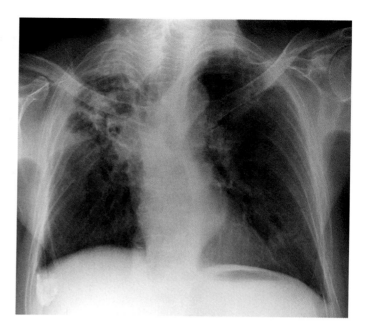

Figure 3.39 Reactivated ('post-primary') tuberculosis with bilateral upper zone infiltration, shrinkage and obvious cavitation. Another hallmark of tuberculosis, namely pleural thickening, is also seen over the lung apices.

CLINICAL CONNECTIONS

In the days when tuberculosis was common, it was well recognized that *Aspergillus* did not colonize active tuberculous cavities – the fungus does not flourish when mycobacteria are present.

The typical radiographic appearances of aspergilloma are those of a cavity filled with a round shadow that represents the fungus ball. This creates the classical 'halo sign' that is illustrated and arrowed in Fig. 3.40. Continued fungus growth may be accompanied by progressive apical pleural thickening over the surface of the colonized cavity and, sometimes, this progressive pleural change is far more impressive than the size of the fungus ball itself.

Primary lung abscess

Primary lung abscess is not common in these days of powerful antibiotics. When it does occur, it may be associated with malignant proximal bronchial obstruction or with alcohol abuse and poor dental hygiene, when, presumably, aspiration is the linking factor. Unusual organisms can be responsible for abscess formation and these include the filamentous bacterium, Actinomyces. The example illustrated in Fig. 3.19 (page 57) was caused by gonococcal infection, the source of which was never identified.

Multiple lung abscesses

Figure 3.41 shows multiple lung abscesses, blood borne from primary pelvic infection. There is obvious cavitation within the largest lesion.

Figure 3.42 is the X-ray of a man who suffered devastating staphylococcal pneumonia following influenza. Amazingly, he survived and his X-ray some years after the acute illness shows scattered micronodular calcification. It is featured in Chapter 4.

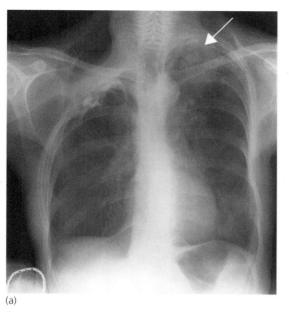

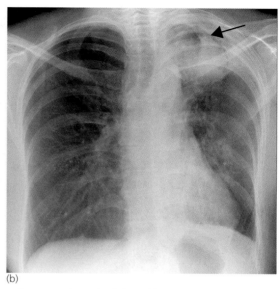

(a)   (b)

Figures 3.40 (a, b) An aspergilloma (mycetoma) at the left apex is present in each of these X-rays and the 'halo' sign is arrowed. This rim of air reflects the presence of the fungus ball within a cavity. Note also the abnormalities at the right apex in (a) with evidence of a previous thoracoplasty and the typical pattern of pleural calcification within an old tuberculous empyema at the right apex.

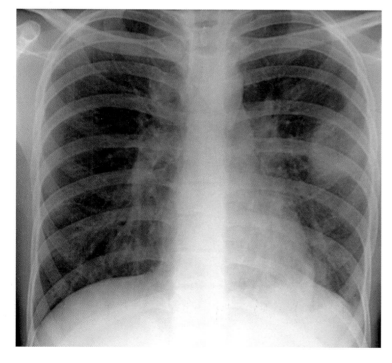

Figure 3.41 Multiple lung abscesses.

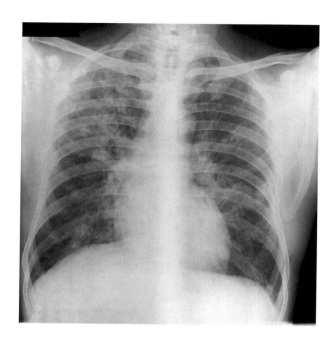

Figure 3.42 Cavitating staphylococcal pneumonia complicating influenza.

Figure 3.43 depicts aggressive tuberculosis in a woman who was immunocompromised by virtue of treatment for extensive carcinoma of the breast. Unhappily, malignant deposits can be seen in the right ribs.

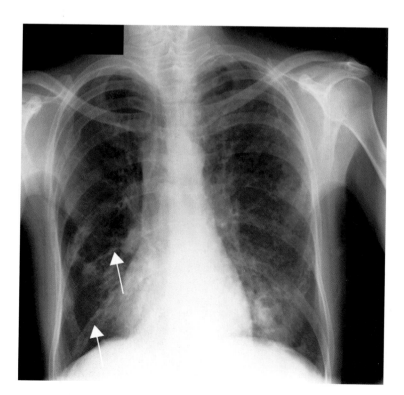

Figure 3.43 Rapidly progressive tuberculosis in a woman undergoing chemotherapy for carcinoma of the breast. Malignant deposits can be seen in several ribs.

Central necrosis

Central necrosis occurs in a number of other pathological processes. Examples are pulmonary infarction, rheumatoid nodules (Fig. 3.44) and progressive massive fibrosis, i.e. complicated coal-worker's pneumoconiosis (Fig. 3.45).

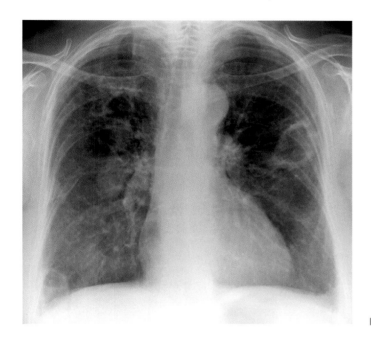

Figure 3.44 Cavitating rheumatoid nodules.

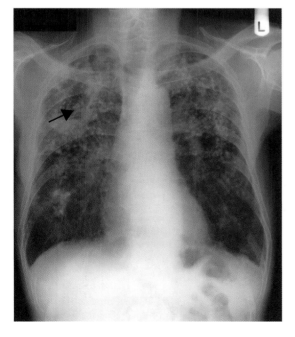

Figure 3.45 This coal miner had circulating rheumatoid factor and the calcified lung lesions are an example of Caplan's syndrome (see Chapter 4, page 108). Cavitation within an area of coalescence of these nodules is arrowed.

Check List Chapter 3

✔ Consolidation occurs when lung tissue is involved in a pathological process that involves air-space (alveolar) filling and the radiographic pattern reflects this.

✔ Consolidation can be confined to a single lobe or segment or be multilobar/multisegmental.

✔ The alveolar space can be invaded by a variety of abnormal exudates/transudates and multiple pathologies can therefore create an identical radiographic appearance. A search should be made for additional X-ray changes that will assist in narrowing the differential diagnosis.

✔ An air bronchogram is created by patent airways becoming surrounded by consolidated lung parenchyma. It will not be present if the pathological process is involving airways as well as the alveolar space.

✔ It is easy to overlook lobar collapse, not least because the shadow created by the abnormal lobe itself may be subtle. There are certain patterns and classical shadows to look for.

✔ Two other groups of radiographic clues are helpful in identifying loss of volume and should be sought proactively:

- 'shift of normal structures'
- 'loss of normal lines and shadows'.

✔ Cavitation is an example of an accompaniment of consolidation that has a specific differential diagnosis.

CHAPTER 4
Pulmonary infiltrates, nodular lesions, ring shadows and calcification

Chapter 3 examined the relationship between the radiographic pattern of alveolar filling and the pathological process of consolidation. It sought to describe an analytical process whereby the differential diagnosis might be narrowed by systematic investigation of details and variations in the basic radiographic pattern. This chapter continues the theme of describing patterns of abnormal intrapulmonary shadowing and attempting to relate them to specific pathological entities – it concentrates on pulmonary infiltrations of various types, cystic shadows and the causes of intrapulmonary calcification. The diversity of abnormal intrapulmonary shadowing presents a huge challenge and is, at first sight, baffling. A fundamental aim of this chapter is to describe a systematic way of unravelling the complexities. Engaging a few simple rules when examining an abnormal pulmonary infiltrate can narrow the differential diagnosis to a few possibilities in many cases and result in a firm diagnosis in a significant proportion.

This approach is based on three lines of questioning:

1. The first asks whether a pulmonary infiltrate is actually present. This can be very difficult to decide when the abnormal shadowing is subtle and a useful arbiter is to question whether the normal vascular pattern is obscured. If it is, then it suggests that abnormal parenchymal shadowing is preventing clear definition of broncho-vascular structures in the lung fields because it has similar radiodensity unlike normal, aerated lung.

2. The second addresses the morphology of the abnormal shadowing.

3. The third concentrates on its distribution.

As with everything else in clinical medicine, there are no absolutes in these definitions and there will certainly be exceptions to the lists of differential diagnoses constructed from this approach. Nevertheless, the technique is useful because it is quick and practical and, most importantly, it is safe. This approach should be combined with other basic observations:

- Are the lung volumes maintained?
- Is cardiomegaly present?
- Are there associated pleural, bony or mediastinal shadows?
- Are there other specific radiographic appearances that give the diagnosis away? An example here is the close association between septal lines and the pathological diagnoses of left heart failure and lymphangitis carcinomatosa.

MORPHOLOGY OF THE SHADOWING WITH DEFINITIONS OF THE DESCRIPTIVE TERMS USED

It is essential to be absolutely clear about the meaning of the descriptive terminology. It is best to describe exactly what you see and avoid over-colourful terminology.

For example, describing a radiographic abnormality as 'honeycombing' is useful provided there is a strict understanding of what is meant by the terminology. The pathological causes of true generalized honeycombing are few and an accurate interpretation of its presence can be diagnostic.

The definitions that follow are fairly standard and, although the measurements quoted are inevitably arbitrary, they are based on years of confirmed practical usefulness. It is important to practise using these terms, to become comfortable with them and to be strict about avoiding vague descriptions that are open to interpretation.

Circular shadows

These are best categorized according to size and all have well-defined borders.

- **Micronodular shadows**. This is my preferred term and is better, I think, than the common synonyms 'pinpoint' or 'fine mottling'. These rounded shadows are small – 1.5 mm or less in diameter).
- **Nodular shadows** are larger, up to 2 cm in diameter.
- **Large circular shadows** are 2 cm or more in diameter.

Ill-defined shadows

This is a descriptive term for poorly defined shadows. They may be reasonably defined and roughly circular or oval in shape, or have irregular boundaries in which case their appearance merges with that of patchy consolidation.

Linear and tubular shadows

Linear shadows vary from 'hair-line' to 2 mm in thickness and include septal lines (see below) and the reticular component of reticulo-nodular shadowing. In his *Principles of Chest X-ray Diagnosis* (1978, Butterworth, London), Simon describes wider band-like shadows as 'tooth-paste' shadows and similar thickness linear shadows with bulbous ends as 'gloved finger' shadows (Fig. 4.1) – both probably represent mucus-filled bronchi. Tubular shadows are described as two more or less parallel fine lines that enclose a radiolucent area and the specific term 'tram-line' shadow can be used when the shadow is the expected size of a bronchus and occurs in a position and with the orientation to be expected of a bronchus. When this applies, the 'tram-line' represents a visible bronchus with thickened walls.

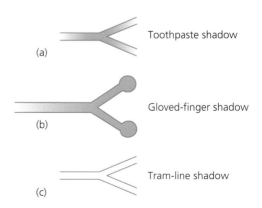

(a)   Toothpaste shadow

(b)   Gloved-finger shadow

(c)   Tram-line shadow

Figure 4.1 Diagram showing 'toothpaste', 'gloved-finger' and 'tubular' shadows (after Simon, G. *Principles of Chest X-ray Diagnosis*, 4th edn, 1978. Butterworth, London).

The terms 'toothpaste', 'gloved-finger' and 'tram-line' are useful not only because the descriptions are clearly recognizable, but also because they point to a specific diagnosis – all three are usually associated with bronchiectasis.

Reticulo-nodular shadowing

The term 'reticulo-nodular' is used to describe a mix of linear and nodular shadowing in varying proportions. The nodular component is usually micronodular or small nodular in size.

Small ring shadows – the honeycomb pattern

I have used this term to describe thin-walled ring shadows each enclosing a relatively radiolucent zone and each measuring up to about 1 cm in diameter.

Larger ring shadows

Large ring shadows are usefully categorized according to two criteria: (1) their diameter; and (2) the thickness of their boundary wall. Bronchogenic cysts and congenital parenchymal cysts present radiographically as large ring shadows with thin walls.

A mycetoma classically presents as a large, thick-walled ring shadow. Cavitation within an area of consolidation can result in very similar appearances and definitions can become blurred under these circumstances.

Septal (interstitial or 'Kerley B' lines (see Fig. 4.2, page 79)

It is worth focusing on these particular linear shadows because they are diagnostically valuable when correctly identified. Septal lines are horizontally orientated, 1–3 mm wide and usually 1–2 cm in length. They are commonly multiple and most are seen in the area above the costophrenic recesses. They are particularly associated with left heart failure, lymphangitis carcinomatosa and coal-worker's pneumoconiosis. The eponymous title, 'Kerley B' lines is commonly used, but I prefer to use the more descriptive terminology.

DISTRIBUTION OF ABNORMAL SHADOWING

The descriptions that follow are intended only as a guide. There are grey areas as far as the distribution patterns themselves are concerned and the differential pathological diagnosis listed against each is not exhaustive. Furthermore, the radiographic appearances of some disease processes are legion and it is almost pointless attempting to fit them into lists: leukaemia, lymphoma and drug-induced infiltrates are typical examples. Despite these qualifications, an attempt to distinguish basic patterns of distribution is a useful exercise in narrowing the disease possibilities for a particular pulmonary infiltrate, particularly when combined with a careful analysis of the component shadows as discussed above.

It is also important to realize that the radiographic appearances of the acute stage of a disease process may be very different from those that are typical of more chronic phases of the same condition – sarcoidosis and extrinsic allergic alveolitis both illustrate this point and examples follow.

CLINICAL CONNECTIONS

The radiographic appearances of sarcoidosis have been usefully categorized into four stages:

- stage 1 refers to hilar and/or mediastinal lymphadenopathy in the absence of pulmonary infiltration
- stage 2 is the concurrent appearance of infiltration and lymphadenopathy
- stage 3 occurs when lymphadenopathy has disappeared but the infiltrate remains
- stage 4 is heralded by the advent of pulmonary fibrosis, usually manifest as upper zone shrinkage and increasing linear shadowing.

There are interesting epidemiological data from Sweden that record the relative frequency of these radiographic stages in individuals presenting with sarcoidosis or found fortuitously to have the disease on radiograph. The prevalence of presentation falls steadily from stage 1 through to stage 4, perhaps suggesting that the stages represent the natural history of the disease, which can spontaneously halt at any stage. Full spontaneous regression of the pulmonary appearance becomes progressively less likely as the stages advance.

There are five schematic distribution patterns to consider and these are shown diagrammatically as reticulo-nodular infiltration in Fig. 4.2.

It is useful to consider these patterns in turn and in relation to the most likely pathological diagnoses that may be expected with each. The categories described below have been subgrouped according to the size of the nodular component.

Mid-zone distribution, with relative apical and basal sparing (Fig. 4.2a)

- Micronodules (<1.5 mm) or small nodules (1.5 mm to 2 cm):
  - sarcoidosis (Figs 4.3 and 4.4)
  - coal-worker's pneumoconiosis (Fig. 4.5)
  - *Pneumocystis carinii* infection (Fig. 4.6).

All zones (Fig. 4.2b)

- Micronodules:
  - miliary tuberculosis (see Fig 3.2, page 47 and Fig. 4.7); in Fig. 3.2, the backgound micronodules can still be distinguished although their profusion resembles widespread consolidation at first sight
  - coal-worker's pneumoconiosis
  - sarcoidosis, a rare appearance (Fig. 4.8).
- Small nodules:
  - pneumoconioses of various types including coal-worker's pneumoconiosis (Fig. 4.9) and silicosis
  - pulmonary metastases, particularly from primary breast or thyroid malignancies (Fig. 4.10)

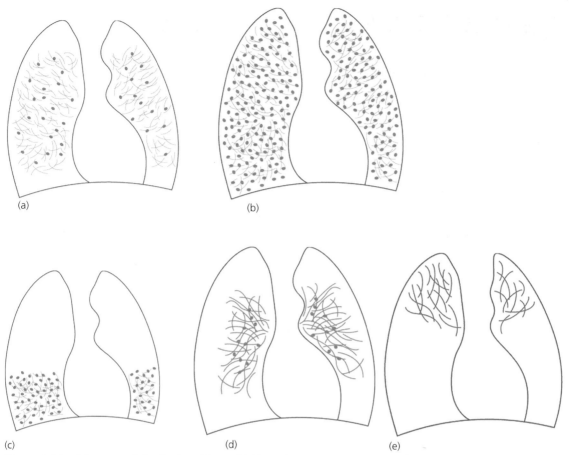

Figure 4.2 (a–e) Patterns of distribution of interstitial lung disease. (a) Relative apical and basal sparing; (b) generalized involvement; (c) predominantly lower zone involvement; (d) peri-hilar predominance; (e) upper zone predominance, often coarse linear shadowing together with upper zone loss of volume.

- sarcoidosis (Fig. 4.11)
- lymphangitis carcinomatosa (Fig. 4.12)
- acute extrinsic allergic alveolitis (Fig. 4.13)
- drug-induced (especially acute reactions, e.g. methotrexate lung – Fig. 4.14)
- lymphoma (Fig. 4.15)
- acute haemosiderosis
- histoplasmosis
- pulmonary eosinophilia (both Loeffler's syndrome and tropical eosinophilia)

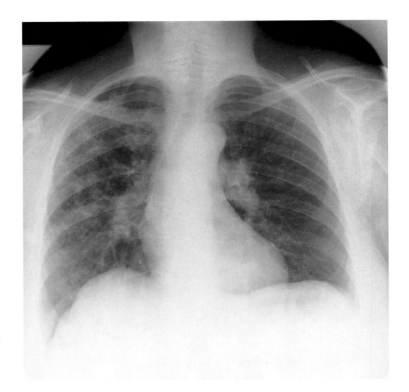

Figure 4.3 Stage 2 sarcoidosis (pulmonary infiltration together with bilateral hilar lymphadenopathy). The infiltrate shows relative apical and basal sparing and the background nodulation is coalescing in areas.

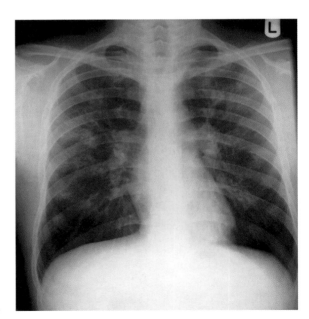

Figure 4.4 Another example of stage 2 sarcoidosis.

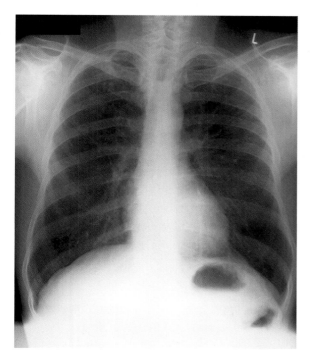

Figure 4.5 Coal-worker's pneumoconiosis. The nodular infiltration in the mid-zones is subtle and the clue to its existence is the blurred outline of the vascular pattern.

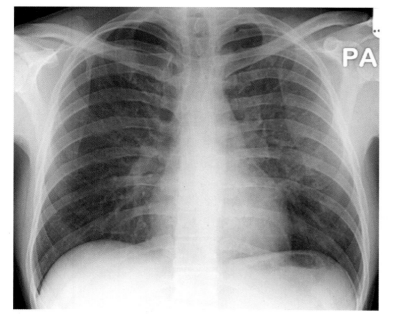

Figure 4.6 *Pneumocystis carinii* pneumonia associated with acquired immunodeficiency syndrome (AIDS). The mid-zone infiltrate is again given away by the obscured vascular pattern.

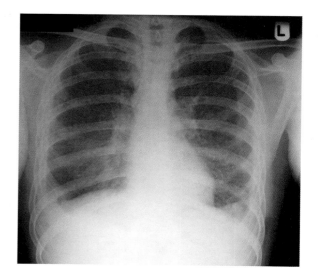

Figure 4.7 Miliary tuberculosis. The micronodules are everywhere, even infiltrating the apices, giving a big clue to the diagnosis.

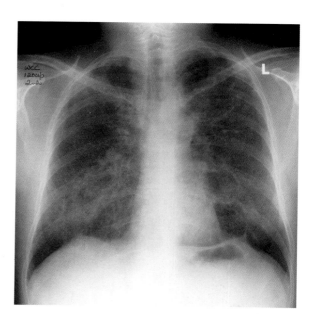

Figure 4.8 Widespread micronodular sarcoidosis is extremely rare and closely mimics miliary tuberculosis.

- lymphangioleiomyomatosis/tuberous sclerosis (the infiltrate is a mix of nodules and micronodules, which may progress to develop classical honeycombing – Fig. 4.16, page 87).
  - Large nodules:
    - pulmonary metastases (Fig. 4.17, page 87).

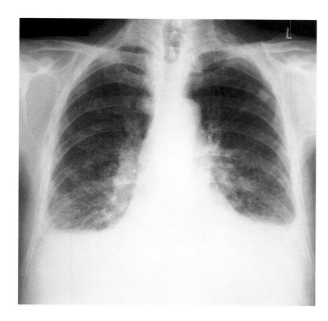

Figure 4.9 Coal-worker's pneumoconiosis. The background nodulation is due to coal-dust deposition. The bilateral pleural effusions developed when this ex-miner developed nephrotic syndrome.

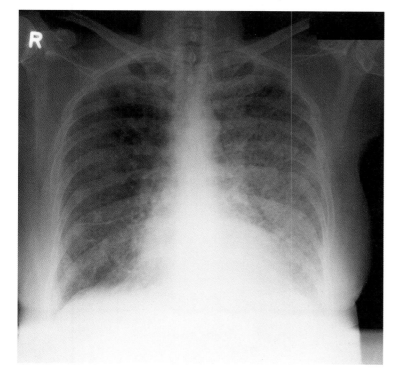

Figure 4.10 Nodular metastases from primary carcinoma of the breast.

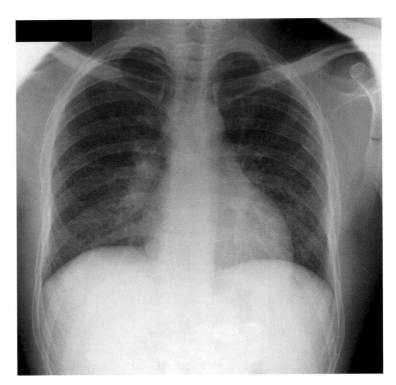

Figure 4.11 Sarcoidosis.

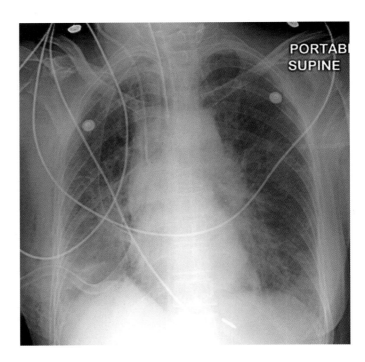

Figure 4.12 Lymphangitis carcinomatosa from a breast primary. The chest drain was required to deal with a large right pleural effusion.

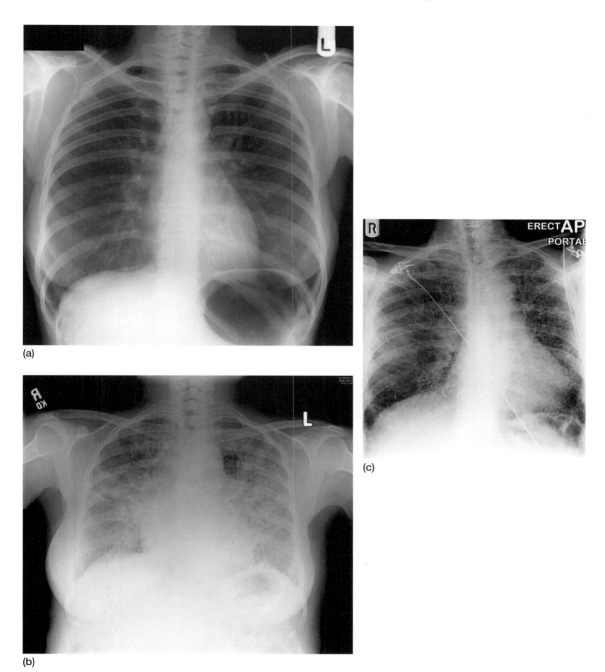

(a)

(b)

(c)

Figure 4.13 (a) Budgerigar fancier's lung. The widespread nodulation is subtle. (b) This was acute, high-dose exposure to bird allergens and the infiltrate is very marked. (c) An example of 'farmer's lung'.

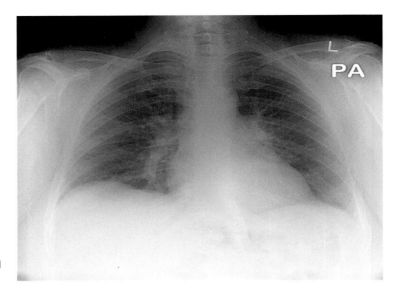

Figure 4.14 Methotrexate-induced pulmonary infiltration.

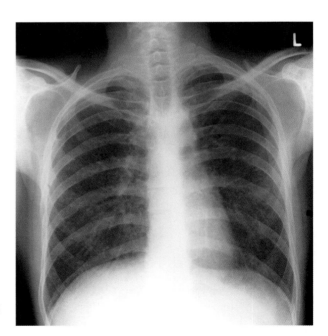

Figure 4.15 Hodgkin's disease with a widespread nodular infiltrate.

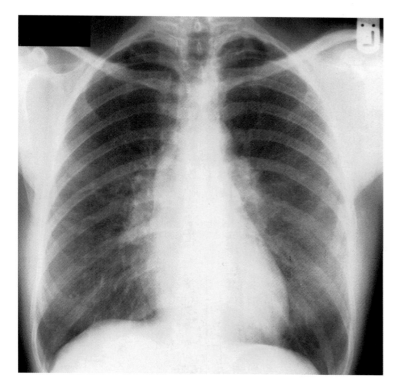

Figure 4.16 Lymphangioleiomyomatosis. This young woman presented with progressive dyspnoea and had severe airflow obstruction. The nodular or micronodular infiltrate is typically accompanied by hyper-expanded lungs (owing to the associated airways obstruction) whereas most infiltrative lung disorders occur in normal size or small lungs.

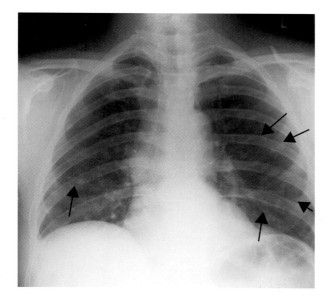

Figure 4.17 Larger nodular metastases from a carcinoma of the bladder.

CLINICAL CONSIDERATIONS

Lymphangioleiomyomatosis. This rare condition is exclusive to women of child-bearing age. The pulmonary infiltrate consists of extensive hamartomatous proliferation of smooth muscle in lung parenchyma, which extends to surround lymphatics, small airways and pulmonary venules. The ensuing obstruction of the respective tissue components results in the complications of chylothorax, recurrent pneumothorax and pulmonary hypertension.

The aetiology may be an imbalance between circulating or tissue oestrogen and progesterone levels and the number of tissue receptors for these hormones, the evidence being as follows:

- the disorder has deteriorated during pregnancy
- progress of the disease slows after the menopause
- oophorectomy and/or progestogen treatment have benefited some patients.

From a radiographic point of view, the appearances are interesting as they show the unusual combination of a progressive pulmonary infiltration in lungs that are increasing in size rather than the opposite.

Predominantly lower zones

- Micronodules:
  - haemosiderosis (chronic).
- Small nodules:
  - cryptogenic fibrosing alveolitis (Figs 4.18–4.20)
  - rheumatoid fibrosing alveolitis
  - collagen vascular disease associated fibrosing alveolitis
  - asbestosis (Fig. 4.21)
  - drug-induced (especially chronic reactions, e.g. bleomycin and busulphan lung).

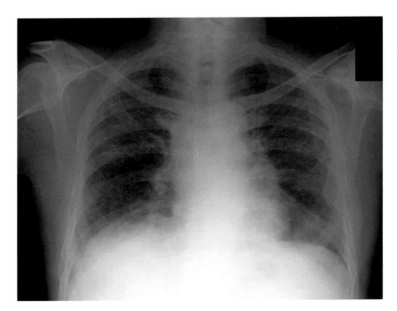

Figure 4.18 Cryptogenic fibrosing alveolitis. The infiltration appears to predominantly lower zone at first but progresses to become more widespread as shown here.

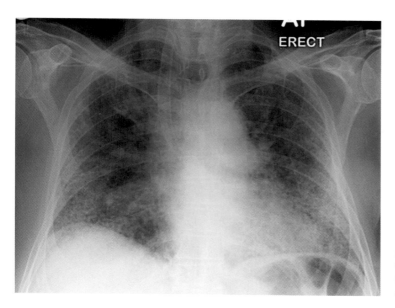

Figure 4.19 Advanced cryptogenic fibrosing alveolitis. Note the small lungs, which had progressively shrunk as the disease progressed.

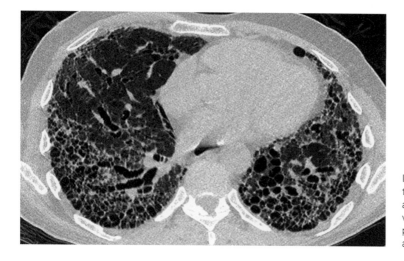

Figure 4.20 This is the computed tomography (CT) scan of Fig. 4.19 and shows the characteristic 'lacework' pattern of the usual interstitial pneumonitis form of fibrosing alveolitis.

Perihilar distribution

- Nodules of varying sizes and often also with confluent shadows:
    - left heart failure (Fig. 4.22)
    - adult respiratory distress syndrome
    - alveolar haemorrhage (e.g. Goodpasture's syndrome) (Fig. 4.23)
    - pulmonary alveolar proteinosis (Fig. 4.24)
    - lymphangitis carcinomatosa
    - *Pneumocystis carinii* pneumonia (Fig. 4.25).

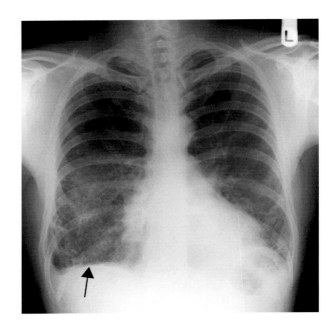

Figure 4.21 Asbestosis. The infiltrate is predominantly lower zone and the diagnosis was given by the accompanying calcified pleural plaque on the right hemidiaphragm (arrowed).

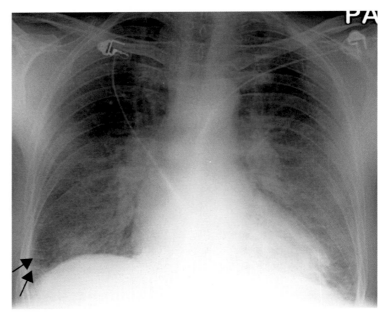

Figure 4.22 Left ventricular failure showing perihilar distribution. The infiltrate is a mix of nodular shadows and an alveolar-filling pattern. Septal lines can be seen at the right base.

Predominantly upper zones (an asterisk indicates association with lung shrinkage and fibrosis)

- Nodules of differing sizes:
  - sarcoidosis* (Fig. 4.26)
  - silicosis*
  - chronic extrinsic allergic alveolitis*
  - ankylosing spondylitis (mainly linear shadows)*

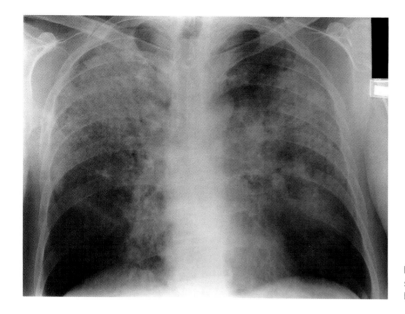

Figure 4.23 Goodpasture's syndrome. Haemoptysis was severe, but this is not always the case.

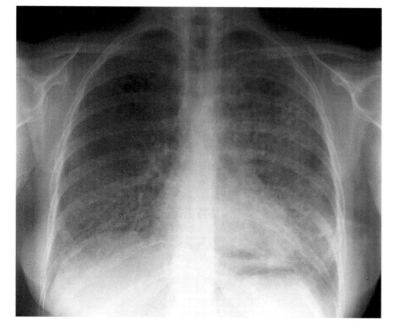

Figure 4.24 Alveolar proteinosis. The appearances are variable in this condition – this patient presented with a nodular perihilar infiltrate, which then progressed to this pattern of more widespread alveolar filling.

- eosinophilic granuloma in its early stages
- post-primary tuberculosis* (see Fig. 3.39, page 70)
- broncho-pulmonary aspergillosis*
- chronic *Klebsiella* pneumonia*
- complicated coal-worker's pneumoconiosis, including progressive massive fibrosis and Caplan's syndrome (Fig. 4.27)
- rheumatoid nodules (Fig. 4.28).

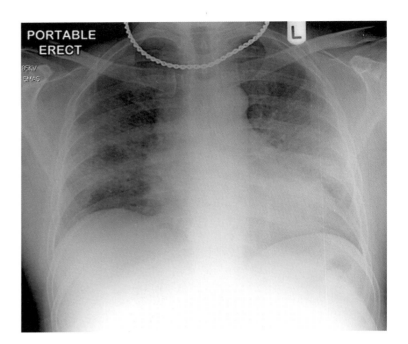

Figure 4.25 *Pneumocystis carinii* pneumonia with a predominantly perihilar distribution.

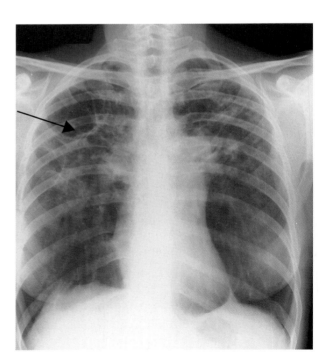

Figure 4.26 Stage 4 sarcoidosis with upper lobe fibrosis and shrinkage. Note the upward movement of both hila. Cavity formation is also seen on the right (arrowed). This appearance is equally compatible with the pulmonary changes of tuberculosis, ankylosing spondylitis and silicosis.

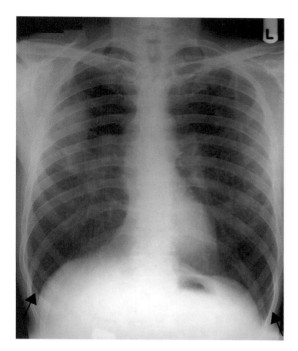

Figure 4.27 Caplan's syndrome. There are nodules up to 1.5 cm diameter in the upper zones and these have coalesced into an area of 'massive fibrosis' on the right. The background dust infiltration is minimal, but septal lines can be seen at the bases.

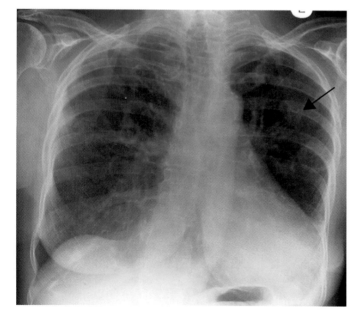

Figure 4.28 Rheumatoid nodules (arrowed).

OTHER PATTERNS OF PULMONARY INFILTRATION

Figure 4.29 shows three other patterns of pulmonary infiltration in diagrammatic form.

Coarse large nodular pattern, often with blurred outline: 'blotchy shadowing'

- Bacterial pneumonia including tuberculosis (Fig. 4.30).
- Non-bacterial pneumonia, for example *Mycoplasma* (Fig. 4.31).
- Viral pneumonia (Fig. 4.32).

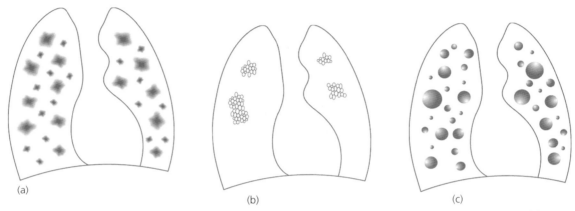

(a)   (b)   (c)

Figure 4.29 (a–c) Three other patterns of intrapulmonary shadowing. (a) Coarse large nodular pattern, often with blurred outlines; (b) 'Honeycombing'; (c) 'Cannonballs'.

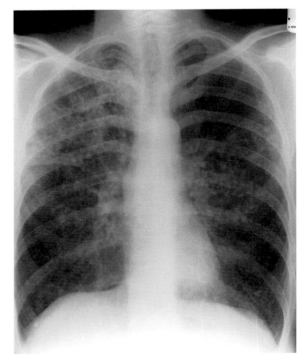

Figure 4.30 Tuberculous bronchopneumonia.

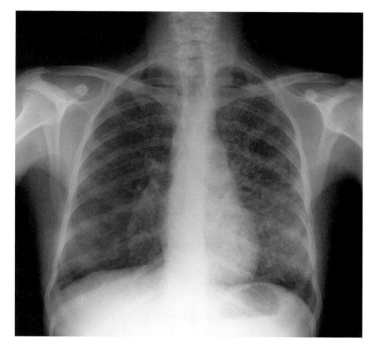

Figure 4.31 *Mycoplasma* pneumonia

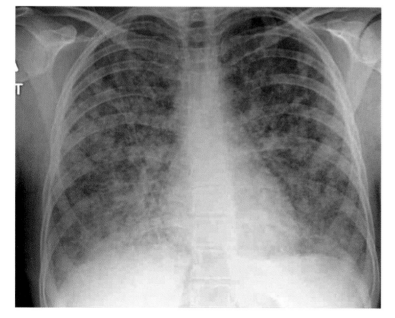

Figure 4.32 Extensive chickenpox pneumonia.

> ### CLINICAL CONNECTIONS
>
> **Non-bacterial pneumonia.** The radiographic appearances of *Mycoplasma pneumonia* vary from typical lobar consolidation to the pattern just illustrated. Clinically, patients can be very sick with fever, tachypnoea and hypoxaemia in association with a dramatically abnormal chest X-ray. Despite this, auscultation of the chest may be surprisingly unimpressive.
> The example illustrating chickenpox pneumonia is extreme. Lung involvement is more pronounced in older individuals with chickenpox and in those who are immunocompromised. The extent of pneumonic change also seems to be proportional to the severity of the skin rash, particularly in adults, and a profuse rash is a useful predictor of pulmonary complications under these circumstances.

- Cystic fibrosis (Fig. 4.33).
- Cryptogenic organizing pneumonitis (Fig. 4.34).
- *Pneumocystis carinii* pneumonia.
- Fungal infection.
- Metastatic malignancies (Fig. 4.35).
- Lung abscesses.
- Vasculitis.
- Lymphoma (Fig. 4.36).
- Drug-induced (Fig. 4.37).

Several examples of diseases producing 'blotchy' pulmonary shadowing follow, illustrating the variability of this appearance. The distinction from patchy

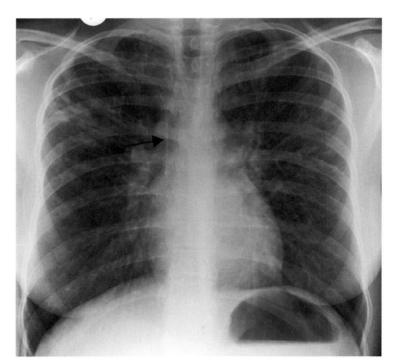

Figure 4.33 A young woman with cystic fibrosis. The central venous line for antibiotic administration is arrowed.

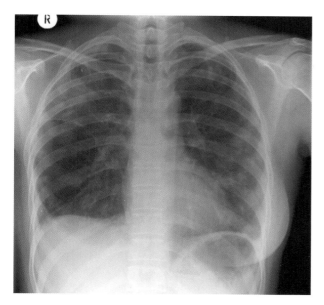

Figure 4.34 An example of cryptogenic organizing pneumonitis.

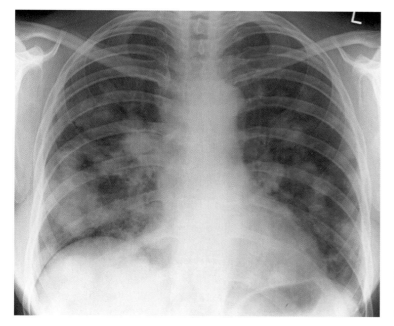

Figure 4.35 Metastases from endometrial carcinoma. The outline of these shadows is not as well defined as classical 'cannon-ball' metastases.

consolidation is blurred but, with many disease processes, one might expect these radiographic appearances to merge one into the other.

Honeycombing

This may be localized, in which case it is seen as a component in many pathological entities including sarcoidosis, fibrosing alveolitis, drug-induced lung disease (Fig. 4.38), extrinsic allergic alveolitis and lymphangitis carcinomatosa.

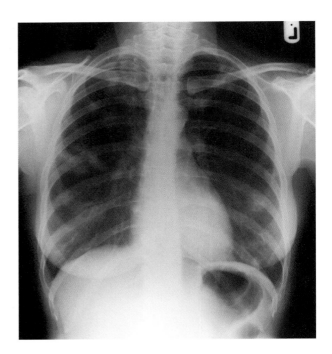

Figure 4.36 Pulmonary involvement in T-cell lymphoma.

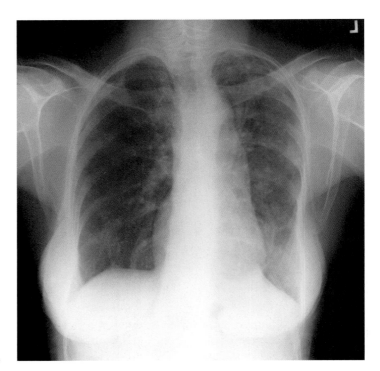

Figure 4.37 'Salazopyrin' lung.

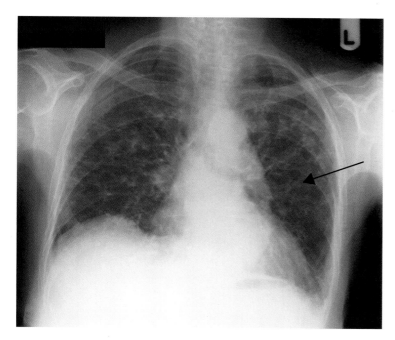

Figure 4.38 'Nitrofurantoin lung' – localized honeycombing is arrowed.

When honeycombing is more extensive the list of possibilities becomes smaller and includes lymphangioleiomyomatosis, tuberous sclerosis and bronchiectasis, although in the latter condition the ring shadows are often thicker walled (Fig. 4.39). The most extreme examples of 'honeycomb lung' are virtually diagnostic of eosinophilic granuloma, a variant of histiocytosis X (Figs 4.40 and 4.41).

Single or multiple, large cystic structures with thin walls may represent emphysematous bullae (see Fig. 1.22, page 16) or congenital, bronchogenic or parenchymal cysts (Fig. 4.42).

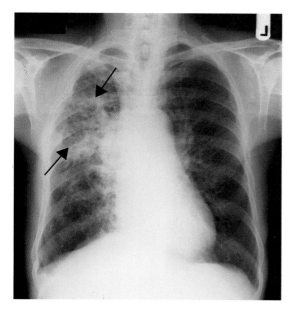

Figure 4.39 Cystic bronchiectasis. The ring shadows are thicker walled.

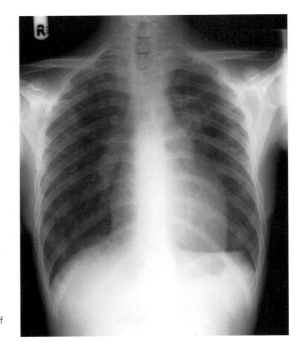

Figure 4.40 Eosinophilic granuloma. A combination of nodular infiltrate and honeycombing is evident.

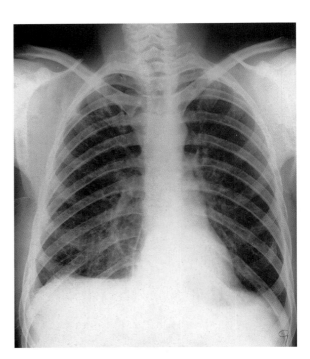

Figure 4.41 Eosinophilic granuloma with widespread, classical honeycombing.

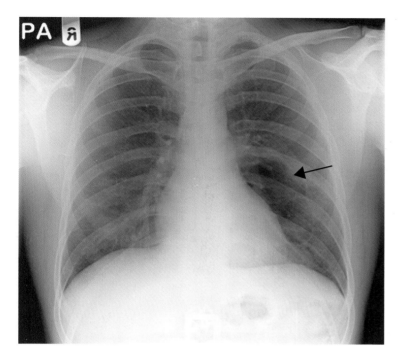

Figure 4.42 A congenital lung cyst (arrowed), adjacent to the left heart border.

'Cannon-balls'

This graphic description of multiple, well-defined rounded shadows of varying sizes is reserved for malignant pulmonary metastases. Although classically described as secondary deposits from carcinomas of the genitourinary tract, they are associated with a diverse selection of primary malignancies (Figs 4.43 and 4.44).

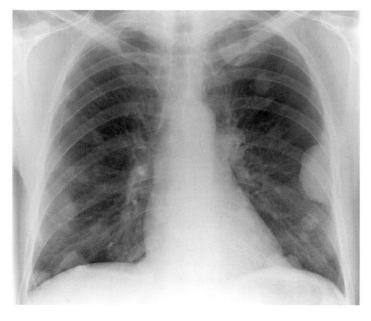

Figure 4.43 Renal carcinoma metastases.

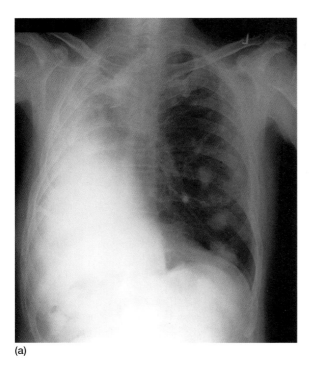

(a)

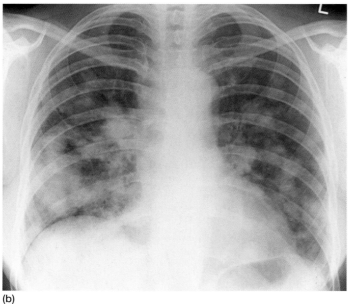

(b)

Figures 4.44 (a, b) Two examples of cannonball metastases from bladder carcinoma. In (a), the 'white-out' of the right hemithorax with mediastinal shift towards the right was as a result of right pneumonectomy for carcinoma of the bronchus several years previously.

THE SOLITARY PULMONARY NODULE

Potential causes of the solitary pulmonary nodule are given in the boxed list. Systematic analysis of the radiograph can narrow the differential but additional imaging and a biopsy are often required for a definitive diagnosis.

PATHOLOGICAL CAUSES OF A PULMONARY NODULE

- Bronchial carcinoma (see Fig. 4.51, page 107)
- Metastasis*
- Granuloma (tuberculosis, sarcoidosis, vasculitis)* (Figs 4.45 and 4.46)
- Hamartoma
- Bronchial adenoma
- Lymphoma*
- Abscess*
- 'Round pneumonia' (Fig. 4.47)
- Rheumatoid nodule*
- Round atelectasis (Figs 4.48 and 4.49)
- Pneumoconiosis (progressive massive fibrosis, Caplan's syndrome)*
- Arteriovenous malformation
- Pulmonary infarct*
- Haematoma
- Fluid-filled cyst or bulla
- Sequestrated lung segment

Notes: An asterisk indicates conditions that commonly cause multiple lesions. The list is not exhaustive; it indicates the commoner possibilities that should be in your differential diagnosis.

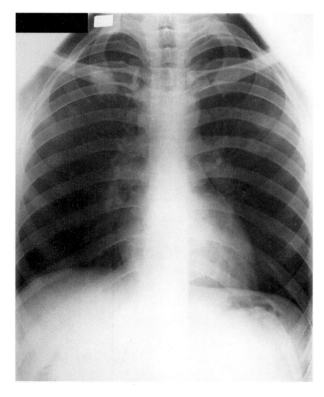

Figure 4.45 Sarcoidosis. The nodule in the right upper zone is clearly seen and there are other, fainter nodules bilaterally.

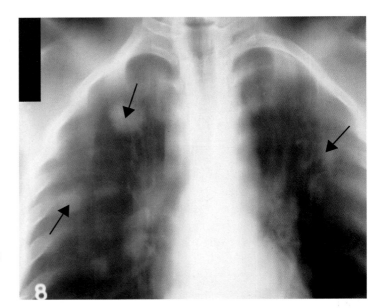

Figure 4.46 The nodules in Fig. 4.45 are clearly shown on old-fashioned tomography. This is an unusual appearance for sarcoidosis.

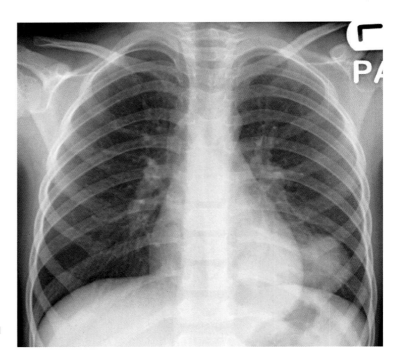

Figure 4.47 The lesion in the left lower lobe is an example of 'round pneumonia'.

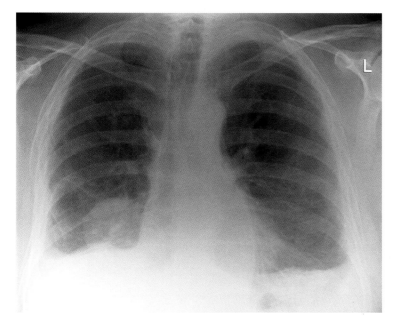

Figure 4.48 Round atelectasis in a 79-year-old man with a history of asbestos exposure.

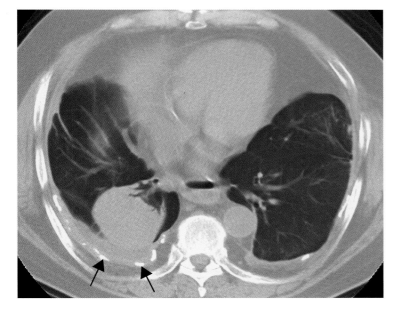

Figure 4.49 A CT image of the patient shown in Fig. 4.48. The intrapulmonary lesion is contiguous with a calcified pleural plaque.

CLINICAL CONNECTIONS

Round pneumonia and round atelectasis. Round pneumonia probably represents an early stage of what will develop into lobar pneumonic consolidation and may represent lung segments that are swollen by contained exudate. It's interesting that this appearance is especially seen in younger people (perhaps their pulmonary architecture is more flexible) and also that it is reported in cases of severe acute respiratory syndrome (SARS), caused by the SARS coronavirus.

Round atelectasis is probably caused by infolding of the pleura and is well recognized in association with asbestos-induced pleural disease.

One systematic approach to radiographic interpretation of the solitary pulmonary nodule is as follows:

1. **Is its margin well defined?** Malignancies tend to be well defined but not exclusively. Other, non-malignant aetiologies can have well-defined borders, for example pulmonary infarction, round pneumonia and round atelectasis.

PEARL OF WISDOM

Particular appearances of malignancy:

- The border of a pulmonary nodule may have an irregular, spiculated or 'thorny' appearance. This appearance has been called the 'corona maligna' (malignant crown) and is highly suggestive of malignant disease.
- Similarly, streaky shadows appearing to link a nodule with the hilar shadow ('the comet's tail') are also highly suspicious of malignancy – they may represent localized lymphatic infiltration.

2. **Has the nodule changed in size rapidly?** Rapid growth usually indicates malignancy. The converse is not reliable as some malignancies can be slow growing.

3. **Does the nodule contain calcium?** In the UK, most calcified nodules are tuberculous in origin. Histoplasmosis is a common cause in endemic areas in the USA and may produce a characteristic 'bull's-eye' appearance with calcium at the centre of the nodule. A hamartoma may display scattered, intralesional ('popcorn') calcification (Fig. 4.50).

HAZARD

Calcification is usually associated with a benign lesion but caution is necessary, for example a granuloma can become complicated by pulmonary malignancy, the so-called 'scar cancer'.

4. **Is the lesion accompanied by significant collapse?** Localized segmental or lobar collapse is suggestive of malignancy as discussed above.

5. **Is there associated pleural, bony or lymph node disease?** All of these features ring alarm bells that the pathology may be malignant (Fig. 4.51).

DIFFUSE INTRAPULMONARY CALCIFICATION

Diffuse pulmonary calcinosis and **diffuse pulmonary ossification** describe the widespread deposition of calcium and bone, respectively, within the lung parenchyma:

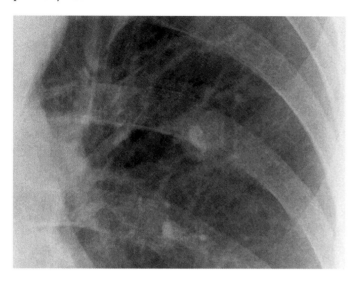

Figure 4.50 Speckled calcification within a hamartoma.

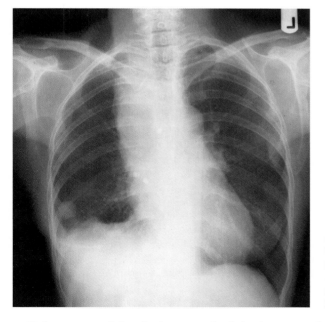

Figure 4.51 An intrapulmonary nodule in the right lower zone was accompanied by right paratracheal lymphadenopathy and a right pleural effusion. Unfortunately, the expected diagnosis of bronchial carcinoma was confirmed by bronchoscopic lung biopsy.

- **Pulmonary calcinosis** is recognized in hyperparathyroidism, chronic renal disease, hypervitaminosis D, pseudoxanthoma elasticum and in association with malignant tumours causing hypercalcaemia.

- **Pulmonary ossification** is usually idiopathic but can complicate intrapulmonary amyloidosis and, when rheumatic heart disease was common, it was seen in association with chronic mitral stenosis.

Both of these diffuse conditions are vanishingly rare, but we do see other causes of intrapulmonary calcification more commonly:

- **Old healed pulmonary tuberculosis.** The calcification may be micronodular or the nodules may vary between 2 and 10 mm in diameter. They may be widespread and, in the case of the miliary (micronodular) pattern, can be identified all the way to the lung apices. Look for associated pleural changes.

- **Previous chicken pox.** The calcified lesions are usually micronodular, often at the bases and not so profuse. They represent healed viral pneumonic change (Fig. 4.52).

- **Industrial lung disease.** Not many of the pneumoconioses calcify. The exceptions are:
  - **Silicosis.** Silica (unlike coal dust) is highly fibrogenic and its early, predominantly mid-zone deposition is readily accompanied by upper-zone shrinkage – look for loss of volume indicated by hilar shadows that are pulled upwards. 'Egg-shell' calcification of the hilar lymph nodes is sometimes also seen.
  - **Caplan's syndrome.** This type of progressive massive fibrosis complicates coal-workers' pneumoconiosis in the presence of circulating rheumatoid factor. Somehow, the combined insult of inhaled dust plus circulating rheumatoid factor conspires to cause this severe form of pulmonary necrosis (see Fig. 4.27, page 93).

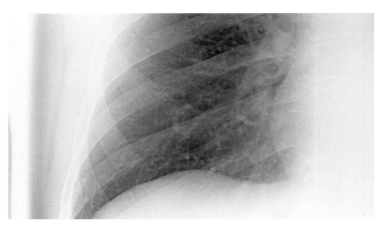

Figure 4.52 Micronodular calcification in the right lower zone following chickenpox pneumonia.

PEARL OF WISDOM

Caplan, a radiologist in Cardiff in the 1950s, described the syndrome that bears his name. He first noticed an association between progressive massive fibrosis and circulating rheumatoid factor and there were two observations that made the miners he described remarkable. The first was the paucity of their background simple pneumoconiosis (usually in progressive massive fibrosis the background nodulation is heavy, reflecting considerable dust deposition in the lungs). The second was the presence of rheumatoid arthritis, the clinical manifestations of which were often mild. It later became clear that clinical arthritis was not always present but circulating rheumatoid factor was. Pathologically, it seems that there is some synergistic interplay between rheumatoid factor and coal dust in initiating lung injury. Caplan also noticed that this variety of progressive massive fibrosis had a proclivity for calcification, whereas 'normal' progressive massive fibrosis did not.

Caplan's original description was of large areas of fibrosis and the story was completed a few years later when he described his 'extended definition' of the syndrome where the nodules were more numerous and smaller (several millimetres to several centimetres in diameter) (Fig. 4.27, page 93). This is a marvellous example of astute radiological observation combined with brilliant clinical detective work.

- **Other radiodense but non-calcific pneumoconioses** include stannosis (tin), siderosis (iron), baritosis (barium) and talc-worker's lung.

CLINICAL CONNECTIONS

The radiographic appearances of barium and iron can diminish if exposure ends and this is due to effective mechanisms for clearance of the dusts. The converse is true with silica, where fibrosis can progress and calcification can occur, even after exposure has ceased.

- **Fungal infections**:
  - **Histoplasmosis.** The major endemic areas for this infection are the great river valleys of North America.
  - **Coccidioidomycosis** can also result in diffuse pulmonary calcification. It is caused by inhalation of a soil-living fungus that thrives in semi-arid conditions. It is endemic from 40° north, 120° west in California to 40° south, 65° west in Argentina.
- **Rarities**:
  - **Osteogenic sarcoma.** Secondary deposits are reported to have been responsible for diffuse intrapulmonary calcification but the likelihood of a patient surviving with such an aggressive primary malignancy for sufficient time to allow the radiographic changes to develop is remote.
  - **Calcification following staphylococcal pneumonia.** This does occur, although rarely. It is not clear whether the phenomenon is caused by staphylococcal infection per se or by the viral pneumonia that may have preceded it (Fig. 4.53).
  - **Pulmonary alveolar microlithiasis.** In this condition of unknown cause, calcified, 'onion-skin' spherical structures are found within alveoli. These lesions can eventually ossify and there is a striking discrepancy between the lack of clinical symptoms and the dramatic radiographic shadowing (Fig. 4.54).

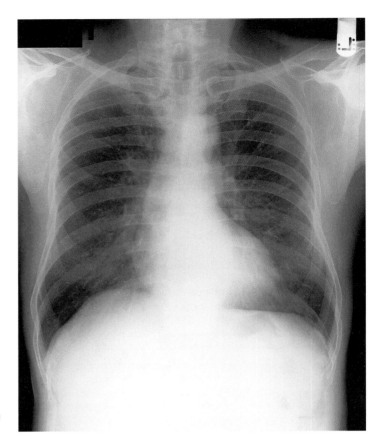

Figure 4.53 Intrapulmonary calcification after staphylococcal pneumonia.

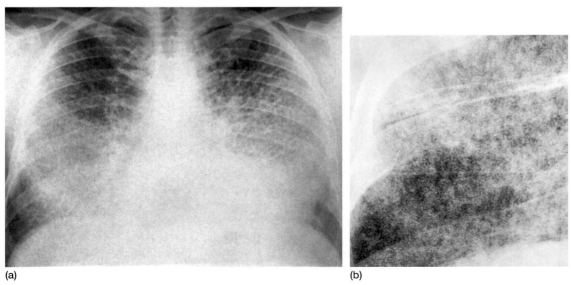

(a)   (b)

Figure 4.54 Pulmonary alveolar microlithiasis (from Fraser RG and Pare JAP. *Diagnosis of Diseases of the Chest*, 2nd edn, vol. 3, 1978. Saunders, Philadelphia).

Check List Chapter 4

✔ **Step 1**. Is an infiltrate present? A major clue is provided by obscurity of the normal broncho-vascular pattern.

✔ **Step 2**. Analyse the type of radiographic shadow that makes up the infiltrate and be careful about terminology. Some recognizable shadows are virtually diagnostic of clinical conditions, for example toothpaste shadows and generalized honeycombing.

✔ **Step 3**. Attempt to identify the distribution of the pulmonary infiltrate into typical patterns.

Combining steps 2 and 3 can help in narrowing the differential diagnosis.

Learn to identify other types of radiographic patterns, including larger areas of infiltrate that may be poorly defined ('blotchy') or well defined (suggestive of malignancy). Marked variation in size of larger, well-defined shadows is also a feature of malignancy ('cannon-balls').

Determining the characteristics of ring shadows and of calcification and knowing the conditions that can be responsible for both is also important.

CHAPTER 5

Pleural disease

Chapters 3 and 4 concentrated on the wide variety of diseases that can affect the lung parenchyma and the diversity of the intrapulmonary shadowing that they cause. Many diseases also involve and invade the pleura but, when they do, the variety of radiographic shadowing that results is limited. This chapter describes the radiographic appearances that result from the presence of air (pneumothorax), fluid (pleural effusion), pus (empyema) and solid tumour within the pleural cavity. Combinations of these 'fillings' occur (e.g. hydropneumothorax and pyopneumothorax) and pleural fluid may be composed of transudate, exudate, blood and, rarely, chyle. There are also characteristic patterns of pleural calcification and these are discussed at the end of the chapter.

The management of pleural disease can be difficult. There are serious potential diagnostic pitfalls and accurate radiographic interpretation is paramount in avoiding these. Clinical management and radiographic diagnosis are intimately interwoven when dealing with pleural disease and this interplay provides much of the emphasis of this chapter. Please note the 'Hazard' icons, highlighting potential mistakes that can have severe clinical consequences.

PNEUMOTHORAX (SEE FIG. 1.21, PAGE 16)

There is a little respiratory physiology to start with because it helps in understanding the management and prognosis of pneumothorax.

Intra-alveolar pressure is greater than intrapleural pressure. It follows that if an alveolus ruptures, air will pass into the pleural space until the pressure equalizes. The pressure changes that occur within the affected hemithorax result in depression of the hemidiaphragm and shift of the mediastinum to the opposite side. If the degree of mediastinal shift is sufficient to compromise the normal lung and/or the rise in intrapleural pressure sufficient to impair venous return to the right side of the heart (and therefore systemic cardiac output) the pneumothorax is said to be under 'tension'. This is a medical emergency – the radiographic hallmark is significant mediastinal shift and the clinical hallmarks are tracheal deviation on palpation in the suprasternal notch and cardiovascular compromise.

> **⚡ HAZARD**
>
> Even relatively small pneumothoraces can result in tension, the reason probably being that the visceral pleura creates a flap over the leak and operates as a ball valve, allowing air to pass into the pleural space on inspiration but preventing its escape during expiration. A dramatic increase in intrapleural pressure can subsequently occur, sometimes with relatively small volume change. **Always check clinically and radiographically for mediastinal shift.**

CLINICAL CONNECTIONS

Once the air leak seals and accumulation of the pneumothorax ceases, re-expansion will take place at a the rate of 1.25 per cent of the volume of the hemithorax per day. This natural reabsorption is speeded by administering oxygen.

Pneumothoraces are either spontaneous or traumatic. Spontaneous pneumothoraces can be primary or secondary depending on the presence or absence of underlying lung disease. Primary spontaneous pneumothorax is a common condition, particularly in young men (the male:female ratio is 3:1). It results from rupture of a surface bleb towards the apex of the lung. Tall people are more prone to developing such blebs as the distance from the apex to the base of their lungs is greater and a more negative intrapleural pressure therefore exists at their lung apices.

A number of conditions predispose to secondary spontaneous pneumothorax. These include, commonly, emphysema and asthma, and also tuberculosis, sarcoidosis, cystic fibrosis and staphylococcal pneumonia (probably as a result of its propensity to cavitate). Uncommon pathologies that are complicated by recurrent pneumothoraces are histiocytosis X, pulmonary neurofibromatosis, lymphangioleiomyomatosis, Ehlers-Danlos and Marfan's syndromes and congenital lung cysts. The patients with eosinophilic granuloma and a congenital lung cyst depicted in Figs 4.41 and 4.42 respectively (pages 100 and 101) each suffered pneumothoraces, recurrent in the first case.

CLINICAL CONNECTIONS

The physiological effects of a pneumothorax are exaggerated in the presence of underlying lung disease, as are the symptoms that the patient experiences. From a management point of view, it follows that the threshold for inserting an intercostal drain is lower in those with underlying lung disease.

A small primary spontaneous pneumothorax probably requires no treatment but the problem lies in the definition of 'small'. Much research effort has been exerted in attempting to provide protocols for the management of pneumothorax, including the relative merits of pleural aspiration and pleural drainage. A detailed discussion is inappropriate here and I refer the reader to the British and American Thoracic Society guidelines. However, factors that do influence invasive management will be the degree of symptomatology and physiological derangement, the presence of underlying lung disease and, in my view, the length of the history (if a lung has been collapsed for a period of time its visceral pleura becomes thickened and less compliant to lung re-expansion).

PEARL OF WISDOM

Catamenial pneumothorax. This condition is associated with intrapleural endometriosis with fragments of endometrial tissue probably finding their way into the pleural space through diaphragmatic defects. The fact that such congenital defects are commoner in the right hemidiaphragm explains why almost all documented cases of catamenial pneumothorax have been right sided. At the onset of menstruation, the endometrial patch breaks down and a pneumothorax results. Consider this diagnostic possibility in a young woman with recurrent pneumothoraces – a history that reveals a connection with menstruation should clinch the diagnosis.

The radiographic appearances do not, of course, help in distinguishing the cause of a pneumothorax unless there is evidence of underlying lung disease. There is little difficulty in recognizing a classical pneumothorax with a rim of air surrounding a partially collapsed lung (see Fig. 1.21, page 16), but small leaks can be challenging as can atypical appearances, with localized or unusual accumulation of air, perhaps because of pre-existing pleural adhesions.

> **⚡ HAZARD**
>
> Before inserting a chest drain, be absolutely certain that any abnormal collection of air is in the pleural space – it is not ideal to insert a drain into a bulla or a lung cyst. If in any doubt, discuss further imaging.

PLEURAL EFFUSION

Table 5.1 lists causes of pleural effusion, categorized according to prevalence and on the basis of their being either a transudate or an exudate.

Table 5.1 Causes of pleural effusion

	Common	Less common
Transudates	Heart failure	Myxoedema
	Cirrhosis of the liver	Sarcoidosis
	Nephrotic syndrome	Peritoneal dialysis
Exudates		
Infection	Bacterial pneumonia	Viral pneumonia
	Tuberculosis	Parasitic pneumonia
Malignancy	Bronchial carcinoma	Mesothelioma
	Secondary malignancy	
Collagen vascular	Rheumatoid disease	
	Systemic lupus erythematosus	
Pulmonary embolism		
Subdiaphragmatic pathology	Subphrenic abscess	Pancreatitis (virtually always left-sided because of the anatomical relations of the lesser sac)
Trauma	Haemothorax	Chylothorax

Radiographic appearances

The classical, radiographic appearance of a pleural effusion is unmistakeable – dependent fluid with a lateral meniscus as it tracks up the chest wall (see Fig. 4.51, page 107 and Fig. 5.1).

However, sometimes it can be difficult to differentiate fluid from pleural thickening and quite often it is tricky to decide where the hemidiaphragm lies on the affected side, an important decision if aspiration and/or biopsy is contemplated.

Subpulmonary collections of fluid (Fig. 5.2), interlobar effusion and loculated fluid also demand special care and this is where ultrasound examination and/or computed tomography (CT) scanning come into their own.

The patient shown in Fig. 5.2 has a subpulmonary pleural effusion and this was confirmed with a right lateral decubitus chest X-ray (taken with the patient lying on his right side) that showed a characteristic rim of fluid lying against the dependent right chest wall.

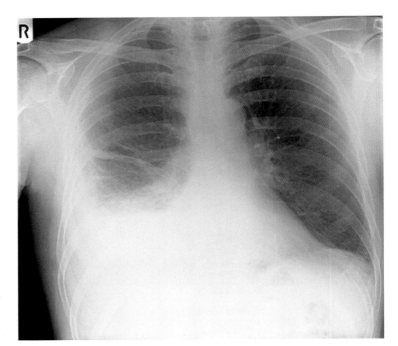

Figure 5.1 Pleural effusion secondary to rheumatoid disease. There is also a nodular pulmonary infiltrate caused by methotrexate.

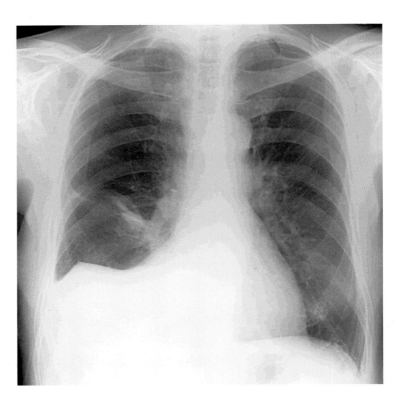

Figure 5.2 A right-sided subpulmonary effusion. The shape of the right hemidiaphragm is very odd and the other clue is the associated fluid in the horizontal fissure. A right lateral decubitus X-ray was diagnostic in the days before ready access to ultrasound and CT scanning.

⚡ HAZARD

Before aspirating or biopsying the pleural space, be certain of the position of the diaphragm. If you are not sure, seek experienced help – a needle in the liver or spleen can have dire consequences.

Size of the effusion and clinical symptoms

The size of an effusion may be helpful diagnostically. In particular, a large collection of fluid (occupying more than 50 per cent of the hemithorax) has relatively few causes. Apart from occasional examples in association with heart failure, pneumonia or pulmonary embolism, the commonest causes of massive effusion are malignancy (lung primary or secondary or mesothelioma), empyema and rheumatoid arthritis.

Clinical features are also helpful. Embolic pleurisy is commonly very painful, as is the pleurisy associated with systemic lupus erythematosus. If an effusion develops in either case it is usually small. In contrast, rheumatoid effusions are usually painless and can be very large. Pleurisy complicating pneumococcal pneumonia is another example of painful accumulation of pleural fluid.

◉ PEARL OF WISDOM

The classical clinical presentation of pneumococcal pneumonia is of a rigor, then fever, quickly followed by pleuritic pain. There is a classic diagnostic catch in that the radiographic abnormalities may lag behind the clinical presentation by several hours. This means that an early radiograph may be normal and the diagnosis can be missed. The clue is the clinical presentation, especially the rigor.

Malignant pleural effusions can be painful but a more common presentation is with breathlessness. Mesothelioma is responsible for both pain and breathlessness and the latter commonly dominates the clinical picture in the early stages when repeated fluid accumulation can be a major problem.

'White-out'

This term describes homogeneous radiodensity of one or other hemithorax. There are four basic causes: total lung collapse, pneumonectomy, consolidation and massive pleural effusion. It is important to determine which of these is responsible and, in particular, to differentiate pleural fluid from the others. A massive pleural effusion will result in a mediastinal shift away from the 'white-out' (Fig. 5.3), whereas lung collapse or pneumonectomy has the opposite effect and tracheal shift will be directed towards the abnormal side (Fig. 5.4 and see Fig. 4.44a, page 102).

⚡ HAZARD

It is vital to differentiate collapse from effusion – inserting an intercostal drain into a collapsed lung can be a fatal mistake.

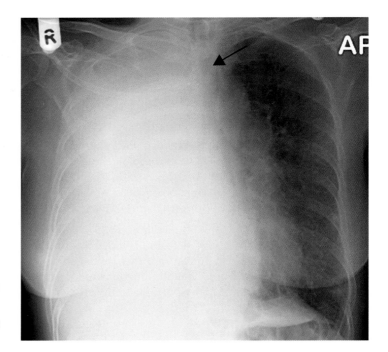

Figure 5.3 White-out of right hemithorax caused by massive pleural effusion. Mediastinal shift, as manifested by tracheal shift, is away from the abnormal side.

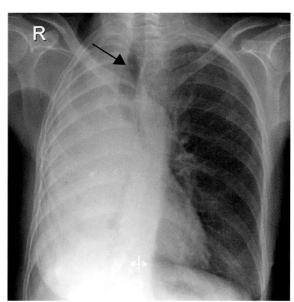

Figure 5.4 Complete collapse of the right lung (carcinoma right main bronchus). In this case, the trachea is directed towards the abnormal side.

Loculation

Loculated pleural fluid tends to be a feature of empyema. It can also occur in other conditions if aspiration or drainage has been partially successful or if fluid re-accumulates after such intervention and pleural adhesions have formed. The natural history of malignant mesothelioma commonly involves the progressive replacement of pleural fluid by solid tumour and the pleural surface often develops a characteristically 'lumpy' appearance.

CLINICAL CONNECTIONS

An empyema requires effective drainage and early liaison between chest physician and surgeon is sensible.

Haemothorax and chylothorax

- **Haemothorax** complicates trauma and this includes iatrogenic trauma. Significantly 'bloody' effusions also occur with malignant conditions and sometimes in association with pulmonary emboli.

- **Chylothorax** results from leakage of chyle from the thoracic duct. This can be congenital due to absence or atresia of the thoracic duct, or acquired following intrathoracic surgery or as a result of non-surgical trauma. The latter are usually penetrating injuries, but chylothorax has been reported after non-penetrating injury, for example hyperextension of the spine or even after violent coughing or vomiting. Finally, non-traumatic chylothorax also occurs and is usually a complication of malignant disease involving the mediastinum.

PEARL OF WISDOM

Chylothorax. Rare, non-traumatic causes include:
- yellow-nail syndrome
- lymphangioleiomyomatosis
- tuberculosis
- filariasis
- thrombosis of the jugular and subclavian veins.

Pleural tumours

Benign pleural fibroma is a rare condition. Figure 5.5 is the chest X-ray of a young woman with lymphangioleiomyomatosis and the lesion on the left proved to be a benign fibroma. I am unaware of any documented association of these two conditions.

Mesothelioma

A thorough industrial history tracing back many years is important when investigating pleural disease. The average latent period between first exposure to asbestos and death from mesothelioma is between 20 and 40 years (in a UK study reported in 1967, a latent period of less than 20 years was uncommon). In addition, the risk of developing mesothelioma is neither proportional to the length nor the heaviness of the reported asbestos exposure.

For obvious reasons, mesothelioma is more common in men. It usually presents with dull chest pain (although pain can be severe and pleuritic) and breathlessness due to the accumulation of pleural fluid. In the later stages of the disease, severe pain may result from invasion of thoracic nerve roots and the tumour also has a proclivity for growing out through the chest wall along the tracks of any instrumentation from aspiration, biopsy or intercostal drainage. This is a very unpleasant complication.

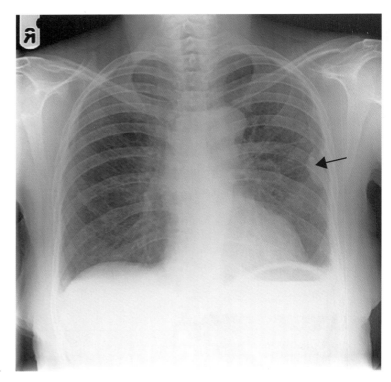

Figure 5.5 Pleural fibroma (arrowed). The background pulmonary infiltrate was due to lymphangioleiomyomatosis.

The chest radiograph usually shows a pleural effusion at first and pleural thickening may be visible above the fluid before or after aspiration. As the tumour progresses, the pleura develops a characteristically lobulated outline (Fig. 5.6) and advanced disease can result in marked contraction of the affected hemithorax. The radiograph

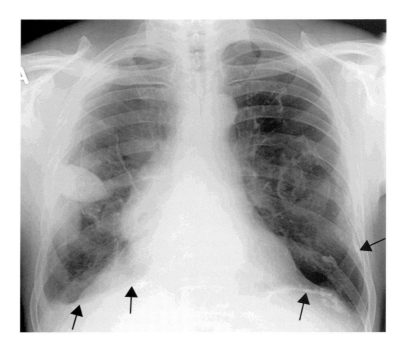

Figure 5.6 The lobulated pleural appearance of right-sided malignant mesothelioma. Calcified pleural plaques are present on the hemidiaphragms and elsewhere.

commonly shows evidence of non-malignant pulmonary or pleural complications of asbestos exposure, as shown in Fig. 5.6.

Secondary tumours

Malignant conditions can, and do, invade the pleura. Figure 5.7 appeared to show an intrapulmonary lesion but turned out to be an expanding bony deposit of malignant myeloma that had destroyed much of the left second rib and was invading the pleura.

Figure 5.8 shows a right-sided pleural effusion accompanied by some solid pleural shadows laterally. The larger, well-defined peripheral shadows on the left are easier to see and all of these pleural abnormalities were caused by secondary invasion from a malignant thymoma, which is arrowed. The primary tumour was occupying the anterior mediastinum and had also spread into the superior compartment, which is quite common for these tumours. The pleural deposits arose as a result of transcoelomic spread from the primary across the pleural space, an unusual but recognized phenomenon with malignant thymic tumours.

PLEURAL CALCIFICATION

There are three main causes of pleural calcification:

- **Calcified asbestos plaques**. The classical 'holly-leaf' pattern of calcification and the typical linear calcified plaques on the hemidiaphragms are both pathognomonic of asbestos plaques (see Figs 1.18 and 1.19 on page 14).

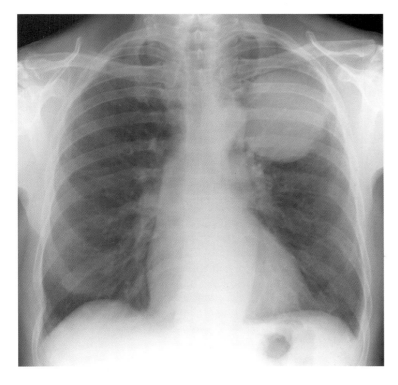

Figure 5.7 A myeloma deposit that has largely destroyed the left second rib and was found to be invading the pleura.

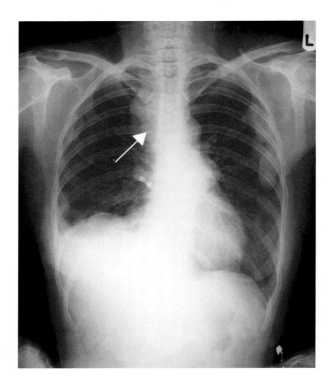

Figure 5.8 Right-sided pleural effusion and bilateral peripheral pleural deposits from a malignant thymoma. The superior mediastinal extension of the tumour is arrowed.

- **Tuberculosis**. Figure 5.9 illustrates another pattern of pleural calcification, this time from an old tuberculous empyema, which is quite different from asbestos pleural disease. The appearances shown in Fig. 5.10 are quite characteristic with a rim of dense calcification outlining the visceral pleura and a network over the anterior and posterior pleural surfaces, seen 'en face' on the postero-anterior (PA) film. This so-called 'en cuirasse' pattern is diagnostic of a previous artificial pneumothorax, a surgical treatment for tuberculosis in the pre-antibiotic era. The calcification arose from the accompanying, healed tuberculous empyema and, for obvious reasons, is rarely seen today. The surgical techniques employed in the era before effective anti-tuberculosis chemotherapy, including artificial pneumothorax, plombage, pneumoperitoneum and especially thoracoplasty, seem quite barbaric now, but they undoubtedly saved many lives in their day.

- **Previous haemothorax**. Figure 5.11 is the radiograph of a man who was a boxer in his younger days. An old healed fracture can just about be made out laterally in the left tenth rib, but the small patch of calcification in the adjacent pleura is clearly seen. Any sort of chest wall trauma can result in this type of pleural calcification but when the appearances are bilateral and multiple, you can be fairly sure that you are looking at the chest radiograph of an ex-boxer.

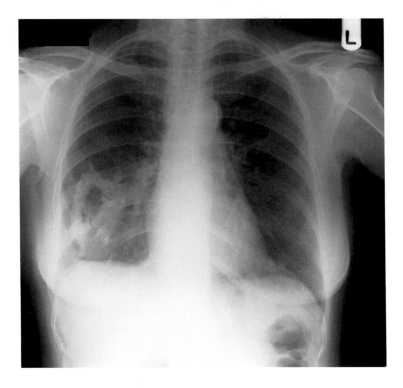

Figure 5.9 Calcification in an old, healed tuberculous empyema.

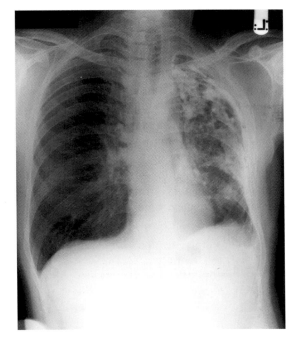

Figure 5.10 The unmistakeable pleural calcification following artificial pneumothorax.

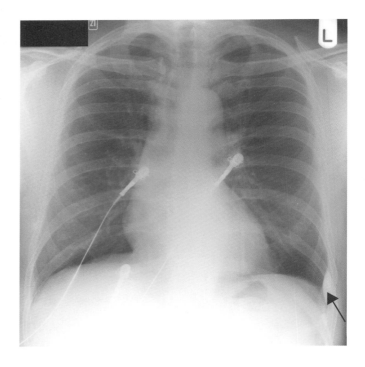

Figure 5.11 Localized pleural calcification (left base) as a result of boxing trauma many years previously.

Check List Chapter 5

✓ Small pneumothoraces may be difficult to spot – look very carefully in anyone presenting with sudden pleuritic chest pain.

✓ If a pneumothorax is present, is there any clinical or radiographic evidence of tension? If so, this is a medical emergency.

✓ Localized pockets of pleural air can be caused by pathology other than localized pneumothorax. The management of a bulla or lung cyst is very different from that of a pneumothorax.

✓ The typical appearance of a pleural effusion is unmistakeable but smaller or loculated collections of fluid (including subpulmonary effusions) are not. Further imaging may be necessary for their exclusion and for guidance before pleural aspiration.

✓ Beware the 'white-out'. It is crucial to establish if this is due to collapse or consolidation rather than pleural fluid. The direction of mediastinal shift provides the clue, but further imaging may be necessary. Do NOT insert a chest drain or even an aspiration needle if you are uncertain.

✓ Pleural shadows may be caused by malignant disease, either primary or secondary.

✓ The patterns of pleural calcification are often diagnostic; asbestos plaques and old tuberculosis are the commonest causes.

CHAPTER 6

The hypoxaemic patient with a normal chest radiograph

Breathlessness is one of the commonest presenting complaints of emergency medical patients and many of them have a normal chest radiograph. These patients deserve considerable thought rather than merely being consigned to the easy diagnostic buckets of 'chest infection' or 'hyperventilation'. A diverse group of medical conditions are capable of causing profound breathlessness without announcing themselves on a chest radiograph and one in particular can prove fatal if undiagnosed.

In this situation, an early step is to ascertain if subjective breathlessness is accompanied by physiological derangement, i.e. hypoxaemia. This cannot be decided simply through arterial oxygen saturation or even with arterial blood gas estimation but only after a thorough analysis of gas exchange. Because of the frequency with which I have seen inadequate assessment of this common clinical scenario, I think it is justified to devote a chapter to its consideration. Anyone dealing with acute medical patients should be aware of the potential diagnoses that explain physiological abnormality (i.e. abnormal gas exchange) in the breathless patient who has no anatomical evidence of disease on his or her chest X-ray. Another justification for including this chapter in a publication that aims to teach X-ray interpretation is that although many of the responsible pathologies are not accompanied by abnormality on the chest X-ray, alternative imaging techniques are far from normal.

This chapter considers three disparate pathological groups: (1) pulmonary vascular disease (particularly of thromboembolic aetiology); (2) airway diseases; and (3) a heterogeneous mix of conditions causing alveolitis, none of which may be detectable on a plain radiograph during the early stages of their natural history.

First, though, it is essential to consider some basic pulmonary physiology in order to follow the diagnostic steps in managing the breathless patient with a normal radiograph.

STEP ONE

Is your patient hypoxaemic as well as breathless? In most emergency departments these days arterial oxygen saturation is a routine measurement and a significant proportion of breathless patients will have arterial blood gases taken as well. However, in my experience, the interpretation of these tests is seldom complete. Let us take an example (a real case) of a 23-year-old, breathless woman whose arterial oxygen saturation (SaO_2) breathing air was 96 per cent.

Can we be completely reassured by the normal oxygen saturation? The answer is 'No' for two reasons. First, the shape of the oxygen dissociation curve means that a SaO_2 of 96 per cent can be achieved with an arterial oxygen tension (paO_2) that may be far from normal in a 23-year-old person. Second, both oxygen saturation and oxygen tension cannot be assessed in isolation because they are both affected by the degree of ventilation – both will increase with increasing ventilation (if the lungs are normal) and hypoventilation will have the opposite effect.

In the example quoted, blood gases were checked, revealing a normal paO_2 at 12.5 kPa, a low arterial carbon dioxide tension ($paCO_2$) of 3 kPa and a pH of 7.49. The low $paCO_2$ indicated that the patient was hyperventilating and, because the paO_2 was normal, primary hyperventilation was diagnosed. This conclusion was dangerously wrong because no objective calculation had been made of the paO_2 that might be expected for the degree of hyperventilation if oxygen exchange was normal.

A fundamental point is that the measured paO_2 is affected by the inspired oxygen concentration (FIO_2) and the degree of alveolar ventilation (VA), as well as the effectiveness or integrity of lung function, which dictates the ability to transfer oxygen from the alveolar space to the pulmonary capillaries.

If lung function is normal, an increase in FIO_2, VA or both will result in an increase in paO_2. A fall in FIO_2 or VA will have the opposite effect. It follows that paO_2 cannot provide an accurate assessment of lung function on its own; it must be examined in relation to what is happening in the alveolar space where the alveolar concentration of oxygen (FAO_2) and therefore its partial pressure (pAO_2), is influenced by both FIO_2 and VA. This young woman's measured arterial carbon dioxide tension ($paCO_2$) was low and, because the transport of carbon dioxide from pulmonary capillary to lung alveolus is highly efficient, we know that her alveolar carbon dioxide tension ($pACO_2$) would have approximated very closely to $paCO_2$ at 3 kPa. Second, the total pressure of alveolar gases must equal atmospheric pressure and if the partial pressure of carbon dioxide in the alveoli falls, the contribution from another gas must rise in order to compensate (otherwise the individual would implode!). The alveolar nitrogen component of inspired air remains constant and so in normal situations this leaves only oxygen to make up for the deficit – in other words, as $pACO_2$ falls, pAO_2 will rise. The opposite is also true; an increase in $pACO_2$ (usually due to hypoventilation) results in a fall in pAO_2.

Going back to the example of the young woman, we are right to infer that a $paCO_2$ of 3 kPa would have resulted in a pAO_2 of more than 12.5 kPa and that her paO_2 should have been correspondingly higher if lung function had been normal. Unlike CO_2, the transfer of oxygen is never perfect (because of an unavoidable degree of ventilation–perfusion mismatch) and this means that there is always an alveolar–arterial oxygen difference ($pAO_2 - paO_2$), which increases with age. Rather than guessing, we should be precise about the paO_2 that can be expected for a particular $paCO_2$ (which reflects the degree of VA) and the first step is to calculate pAO_2. This is straightforward because pAO_2 is easy to calculate using the modified alveolar gas equation as follows:

$$pAO_2 = pIO_2 - \frac{paCO_2}{R}$$

where R is the respiratory quotient (0.8 under most conditions) and pIO_2 is 21 per cent of atmospheric pressure (101 kPa). Saturated water vapour pressure is 6.5 kPa and therefore the partial pressure of oxygen in inspired air is 21 per cent of 94.5 kPa, i.e. 19.845 kPa (or 20 for simplicity).

If we return to the example quoted:

$$pAO_2 = 20 - \frac{3}{0.8}$$

i.e. $pAO_2 = 16.25\,kPa$

Blood gases measure paO_2 and the alveolar–arterial oxygen difference ($pAO_2 - paO_2$) can therefore be calculated and compared with normal values:

$pAO_2 - paO_2 = 16.25 - 12.5 = 3.75\,kPa$.

$pAO_2 - paO_2$ correlates with the degree of ventilation–perfusion mismatch and therefore provides direct information on the integrity of lung function. A gradient of more than 2 kPa is very questionable in a 23 year old and one of 3.75 is definitely abnormal. In other words, by completing this simple calculation, we have shown that the patient is hyperventilating in order to compensate for abnormal oxygen exchange and to avoid hypoxaemia. This is not primary hyperventilation, there is something wrong with her lung function. Moreover, the abnormal physiology is not matched by any pathology that is visible on the chest radiograph and this discrepancy has to be explained.

CLINICAL CONNECTIONS

The above equation is 'modified' because it ignores the fact that we consume a larger volume of oxygen than we produce carbon dioxide. Therefore, with each respiratory cycle the inspired volume of alveolar gas is slightly greater than the expired volume and this is reflected in the full alveolar gas equation. However, the full equation is much more complicated and, in practice, when calculating pAO_2 using the modified method, the inherent error is only a fraction of a kilopascal (kPa) and can be ignored in most clinical situations.

Calculating alveolar oxygen tension in this way becomes increasingly less reliable as the inspired oxygen tension increases. The patient should be breathing air to allow a meaningful calculation, but do not take a hypoxaemic patient off oxygen just to calculate the $pAO_2 - paO_2$ gradient – this is not just pointless, it is dangerous.

Ventilation–perfusion mismatch and its correlate, the $pAO_2 - paO_2$ gradient, both increase with age. A rough estimate of normal values at different ages is given by the equation first described by Mellemgaard et al. in the 1960s:

$$pAO_2 - paO_2 = 2.5 + (\text{age in years} \times 0.21)$$

STEP TWO

This is a short but important step. Consider alternative blood gases in a young man: paO_2 16.5 kPa, $paCO_2$ 2 kPa, pH 7.37

The A–a gradient calculates out at 1 kPa, which is completely normal. The patient is definitely hyperventilating and his lung function is good. However, before diagnosing primary hyperventilation, the parameters of acid–base balance must be examined. This was a real example in a 19-year-old man who had taken a salicylate overdose and was hyperventilating in order to correct for a metabolic acidaemia. The fall in $paCO_2$ as a result of his hyperventilation had largely compensated for the metabolic acidaemia but the measured standard base excess was highly abnormal at −9. The message is: look at all the parameters of acid–base balance, especially those that equate to metabolic disturbance and exclude the effects of ventilatory compensation.

STEP THREE: PULMONARY VASCULAR DISEASE

Let us move on to consider the differential diagnosis in a patient who is breathless and has an abnormal alveolar–arterial oxygen difference with no obvious explanation for this on their chest radiograph.

Figure 6.1 is the chest X-ray of a 60-year-old woman who was referred one evening with a history of sudden onset of breathlessness. She had an A–a gradient of 8 kPa, was breathless at rest and very frightened. There were no abnormal respiratory findings on examination and her radiograph was normal. She was anticoagulated and a computed tomography pulmonary angiogram (CTPA) was requested. Figure 6.2 shows one of the resulting images with thrombus clearly visible in both pulmonary arteries.

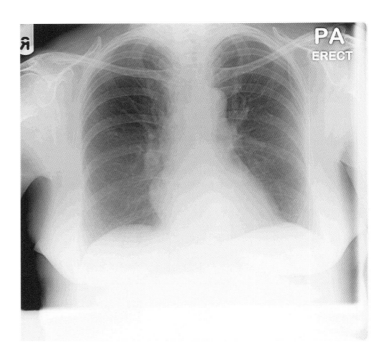

Figure 6.1 Chest X-ray of a 60-year-old woman presenting with sudden dyspnoea.

Major pulmonary embolism can present with minimal abnormal clinical findings, a normal chest X-ray and a blameless electrocardiogram. The basic message is to question the possibility of pulmonary embolism in a patient with abnormal gas exchange (an abnormal $pAO_2 - paO_2$ difference or hypoxaemia) even when the chest X-ray is normal. Pulmonary thrombo-embolic disease is potentially fatal and if one embolism has occurred there may be another one waiting to happen.

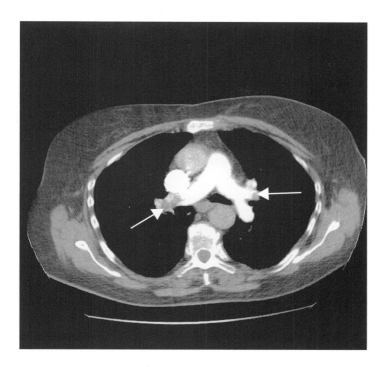

Figure 6.2 CTPA image of the same patient – bilateral thrombus is arrowed.

CLINICAL CONNECTIONS

Pleurisy:

- Smaller pulmonary emboli tend to present with pleurisy perhaps because they are able to reach the periphery of the lung and involve the visceral pleura.
- Large emboli, on the other hand, are regularly painless and present with breathlessness and/or haemodynamic abnormalities.
- The absence of pleurisy does not exclude pulmonary embolism.

Physical signs:

- Quite commonly, there are no abnormal findings especially when the embolism is relatively small.
- An increased respiratory rate may be the only abnormal finding.
- Signs of pulmonary hypertension – elevated jugular venous pressure (perhaps with a prominent 'a' wave), a loud pulmonary second heart sound and a right parasternal heave indicative of right ventricular hypertrophy.
- Large emboli can be accompanied by evidence of compromised systemic cardiac output with hypotension and cold, clammy peripheries.

The abnormal radiograph in pulmonary embolism

There are radiographic abnormalities that accompany pulmonary embolism and some of these are subtle:

- one or other (and occasionally both) hemidiaphragms may be elevated
- there may be line shadows at the bases
- occasionally, a wedge-shaped shadow may be seen with its base adjacent to the pleural surface.

Figure 6.3 illustrates all of these three appearances – a combination that is very unusual.

In addition:

- one or other main pulmonary artery may be bulky, directly reflecting the presence of clot within it
- this 'bulkiness' may be accompanied by Westermark's sign, which describes an area of hypoperfusion somewhere in the lung fields – Fig. 6.4 (a, b) shows examples of this uncommon appearance and the accompanying bulkiness of the right hilum is particularly seen in Fig. 6.4(b).

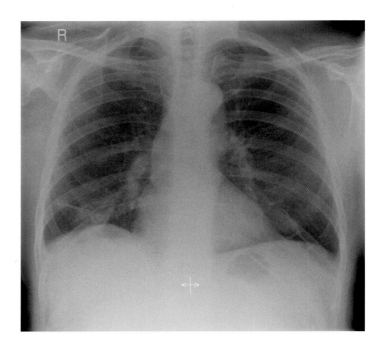

Figure 6.3 Raised right hemidiaphragm, line shadow at the right lower zone and a wedge-shaped shadow based on the pleura at the right base. It is very unusual to see all of these suggestive abnormalities in pulmonary embolism on the same chest X-ray.

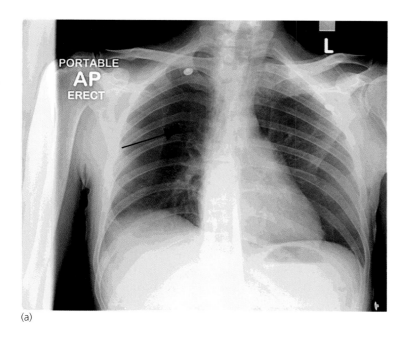

(a)

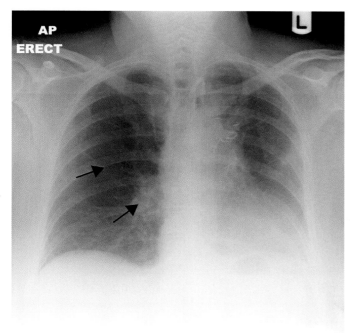

(b)

Figure 6.4 (a, b) Examples of Westermark's sign with areas of hypoperfusion (arrowed). The right hilum is also 'bulky', particularly in Fig. 6.4(b).

Figure 6.5 (a, b) shows computed tomography (CT) slices relating to the previous chest X-rays – thrombus can be seen in both pulmonary arteries. Thrombolysis resulted in excellent resolution of these changes and full clinical recovery.

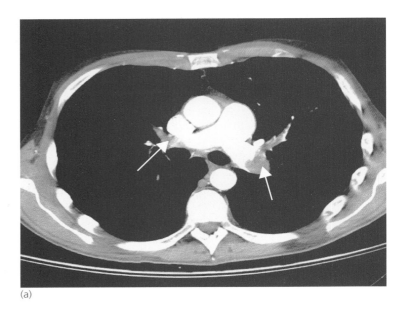

(a)

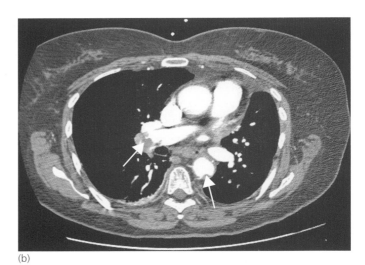

(b)

Figure 6.5 (a, b) CTPA image of the same patients with pulmonary arterial thrombus arrowed.

Other types of pulmonary vascular disease

- **Secondary pulmonary hypertension** often occurs as a result of chronic obstructive pulmonary disease. The cardinal radiographic appearances are those of bilateral enlargement of proximal pulmonary arteries and peripheral vascular attenuation. There may be additional radiographic evidence of disease – for example, see the bulla illustrated in Fig. 1.24 (page 17).

- **Idiopathic pulmonary hypertension** produces the same vascular appearances. Clinically, the presentation tends to be one of progressive, rather than acute, dyspnoea.

STEP FOUR: AIRWAY DISEASES

Diseases predominantly affecting airways commonly cause breathlessness accompanied by abnormal gas exchange. These diseases may not produce radiographic abnormalities. Examples are:

- **Asthma.** Asthmatic patients can be severely hypoxaemic with nothing to show on the radiograph. There is usually no difficulty with diagnosis because the physical findings are quite obvious. The challenge is to recognize just how severe the attack is and objective measurements, especially those of gas exchange, are vital.

- **Smoking-related airways obstruction.** Chronic bronchitis and emphysema also disrupt the ventilation–perfusion relationship and although radiographic abnormalities may be seen (bullae, abnormal vascular distribution or evidence of pulmonary hypertension) the chest X-ray is often unremarkable. Acute infective exacerbation of chronic obstructive pulmonary disease results in further ventilation–perfusion mismatch with consequent further deterioration in hypoxaemia; however, remember that this group of patients is also at risk of pulmonary embolism and that there is no equation that provides a correlation between smoking years and the ensuing disruption to lung function.

- **Acute bronchiolitis.** Well recognized in children, bronchiolitis also affects adults. A variety of common viruses may be responsible and the clinical findings are of a breathless patient, perhaps pyrexial, with a history suggestive of respiratory tract infection and who may be severely hypoxaemic despite having a normal chest X-ray. If physical signs are present these are commonly inspiratory crackles, although high-pitched wheezes ('squawks') may also be found on auscultation.

- **Other airway diseases.** Figures 6.6 and 6.7 illustrate an example of obliterative bronchiolitis. This is a rare condition associated with rheumatoid arthritis and other collagen vascular diseases, although apparently idiopathic in this case. The chest X-ray does show a degree of hyperinflation but the accompanying severe hypoxaemia appeared to be out of proportion to the radiographic change. Figure 6.7 is a CT image taken in expiration showing marked air trapping in lung parenchyma (arrowed).

STEP FIVE: ALVEOLITIDES

Finally, various conditions that result in alveolitis or an alveolar-filling process can cause dramatic disruption to gas exchange despite an apparently normal chest X-ray. A comprehensive history is often the clue and some examples follow:

- Figure 6.8 is a CT image of a 68-year-old woman with rheumatoid arthritis. The CT scan was requested in view of her history of methotrexate therapy and is highly abnormal. This is 'methotrexate lung' and the pulmonary infiltration disappeared following corticosteroid treatment.

- Figure 6.9 shows a 'ground-glass' appearance on CT scan in a 30-year-old farmer. This example of 'farmer's lung' (a type of extrinsic allergic alveolitis) also responded to corticosteroids.

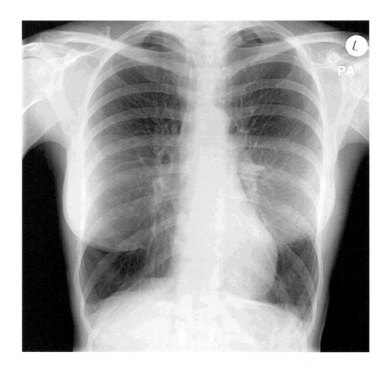

Figure 6.6 A young woman with obliterative bronchiolitis.

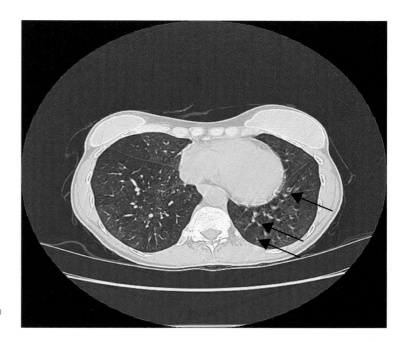

Figure 6.7 CT image of the patient in Fig. 6.6 showing severe air-trapping.

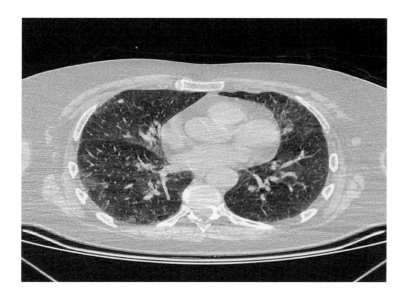

Figure 6.8 Methotrexate lung.

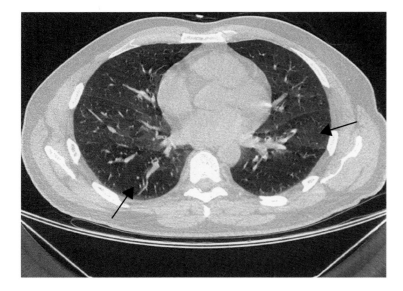

Figure 6.9 Farmer's lung.

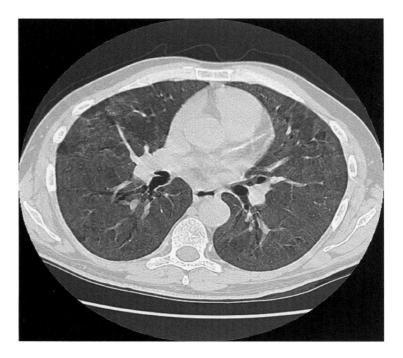

Figure 6.10 Bird-fancier's lung.

- Figure 6.10 is another example of extrinsic allergic alveolitis – in this case 'bird-fancier's lung in a young man who had a parakeet as an indoor pet.

In each of these three examples, 'ground glass' shadowing is seen occupying the lung parenchyma (arrowed in Fig. 6.9).

- *Pneumocystis carinii* pneumonia is well documented as presenting with dyspnoea and (often severe) hypoxia in the presence of a normal or near-normal chest radiograph. The same is also occasionally true of the desquamative form of cryptogenic fibrosing alveolitis.

CHAPTER 7

Practice examples and 'fascinomas'

The final chapter consists of two sections. For the first, I have collected a series of chest radiographs on which to practise the diagnostic skills described so far. The concluding section contains some fascinating radiographs encountered over the years. Although 'fascinomas', by definition, are rare and you may never come across an example yourself in clinical practice, these radiographs are, I believe, instructive in their own right and illustrate the power of systematic observation – one of the basic themes of this book.

PRACTICE EXAMPLES

Examine the radiographs that follow – each of them is accompanied by short clinical notes in the legend. Follow the investigative approach described in earlier chapters, take time to record all of the abnormalities and then make an attempt at a diagnosis. Your observations and conclusions can be checked with the answers that follow.

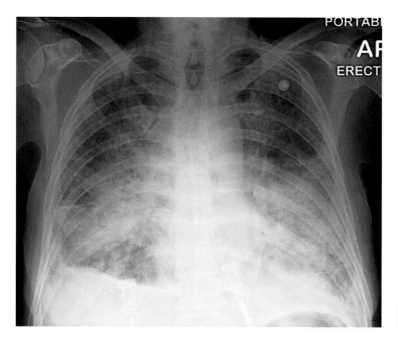

Figure 7.1 This man was admitted to hospital with severe breathlessness.

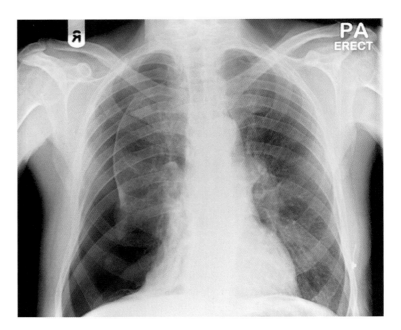

Figure 7.2 Take time to collect all of the information. Then look at Figs 7.3 and 7.4.

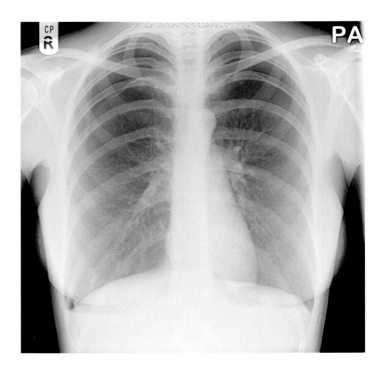

Figure 7.3 This young woman presented with breathlessness and chest pain.

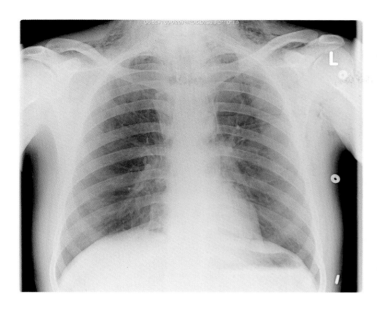

Figure 7.4 This young man was wheezy and breathless.

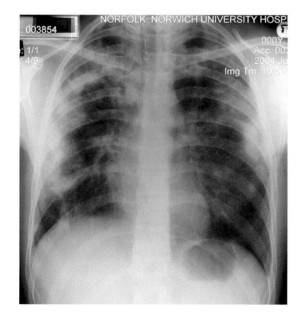

Figure 7.5 This young man had been unwell for 2 weeks before this radiograph was taken. His symptoms were fever, cough and severe general malaise. Note the distribution of the abnormal pulmonary shadowing.

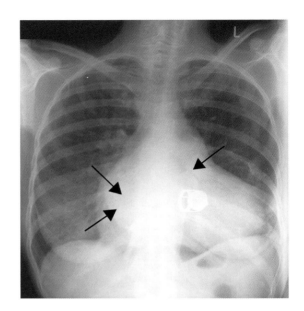

Figure 7.6 There are lots of abnormalities on this radiograph and they come together to tell quite a story about this woman who suffered rheumatic fever in childhood.

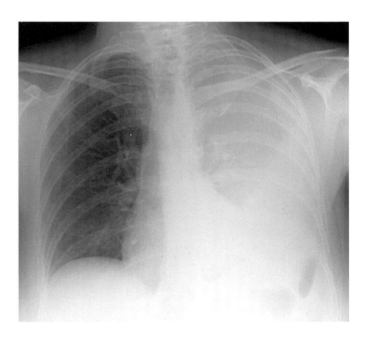

Figure 7.7 Weight loss and fever were the presenting complaints and this woman was severely cachectic when she finally came to hospital. How will you manage the problem?

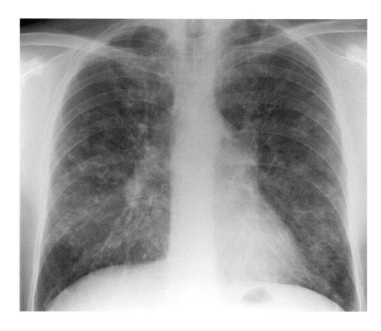

Figure 7.8 This 19 year old had been under the care of the chest clinic since early childhood.

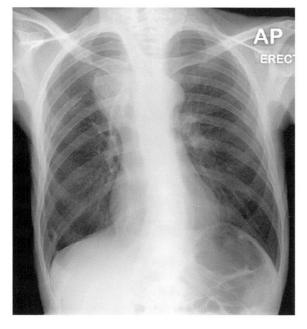

Figure 7.9 This young man presented with weight loss and chest pain when imbibing alcohol.

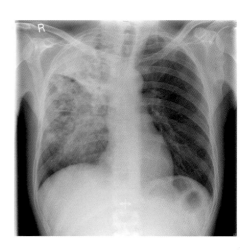

Figure 7.10 The presenting complaints were night sweats and weight loss in both of these patients. Describe the radiographic abnormalities in each X-ray. What is the most likely diagnosis?

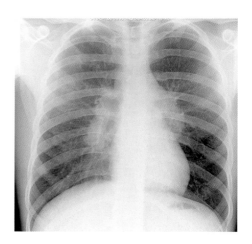

Figure 7.11 The combination of mediastinal and parenchymal lung abnormalities should suggest a particular diagnosis. How do you think this patient (who was in his twenties) might have presented?

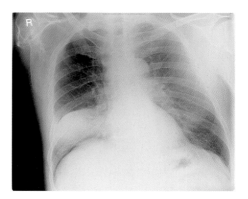

Figure 7.12 The radiographic abnormalities are a mix of old and new. What do you see altogether?

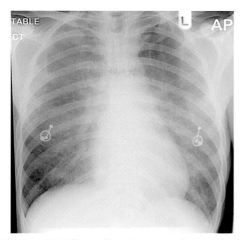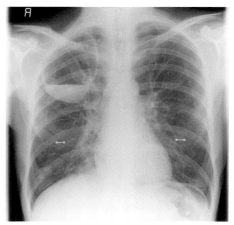

Figures 7.13 and 7.14 These films have one abnormality in common. What is it? The lung pathologies are very different. Describe what you see in both cases. How may the underlying pathology be linked in these two patients?

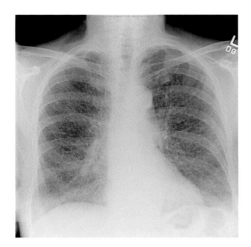

Figure 7.15 Describe the pulmonary infiltrate. What is your differential diagnosis?

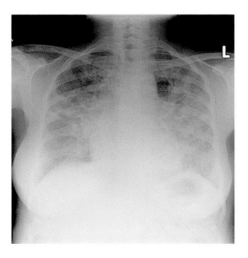

Figure 7.16 Here is another pulmonary infiltrate. Describe the nature of the shadowing and its distribution.

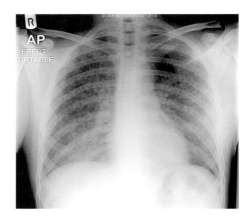

Figure 7.17 Yet another pulmonary infiltrate to practise on.

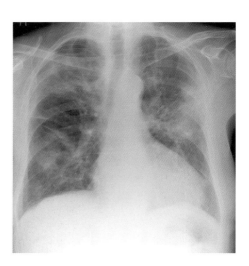

Figure 7.18 The parenchymal lung appearances are quite different here. Just describe what you see and suggest some diagnoses. This was a very unusual case.

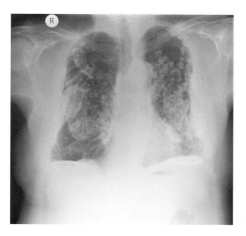

Figure 7.19 These are classical appearances. What is the diagnosis and why?

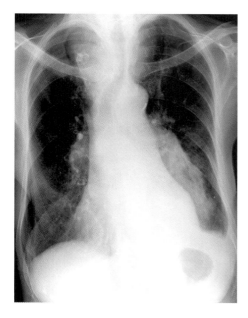

Figure 7.20 This elderly woman has a large mass in the left lower zone which proved to be a carcinoma of the bronchus. There is another abnormality, what is it?

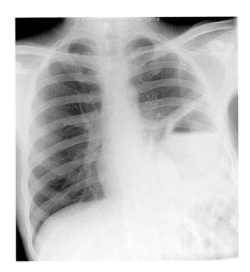

Figure 7.21 Describe the abnormalities. What is the likely diagnosis? How would you manage this problem?

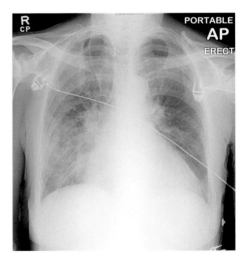

Figure 7.22 Use the systematic approach to list all of the abnormal findings here.

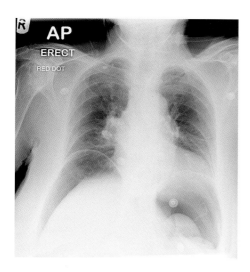

Figure 7.23 There is more than one abnormality on this film also.

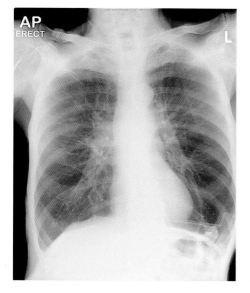

Figure 7.24 This middle-aged patient was extremely breathless and hypoxic on admission.

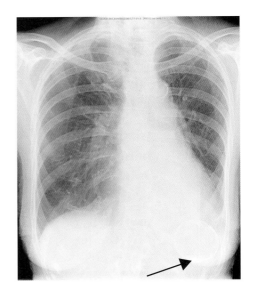

Figure 7.25 What structures are calcified?

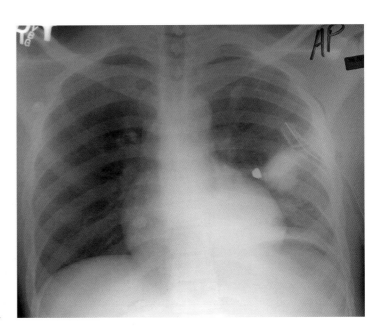

Figure 7.26 Have a shot at this diagnosis.

ANSWERS

- **Figure 7.1**. Pulmonary infiltration is perihilar in distribution and has coalesced to produce an alveolar-filling pattern. This is an antero-posterior (AP) film and it is impossible to comment on heart size but there is pleural fluid, certainly on the right. The intrapulmonary shadowing is too dense to see septal lines, but the most likely diagnosis is left ventricular failure. However, other possibilities exist, including alveolar haemorrhage, adult respiratory distress syndrome, pneumocystis pneumonia and pulmonary alveolar proteinosis.

- **Figure 7.2**. This shows a large right-sided pneumothorax and the right lower lobe is completely collapsed (diagonal shadow adjacent to right heart border). The proximal pulmonary vessels are prominent and this was a secondary pneumothorax in a man who had been a life-long heavy smoker.

- **Figure 7.3**. This shows bilateral pneumothoraces in a young woman (note the breast shadows). Spontaneous pneumothoraces are possible of course, particularly if she was tall and thin, but consider possible underlying pathology in a young woman – catamenial pneumothorax is unlikely as these are bilateral and there was a primary lung problem in the form of lymphangioleiomyomatosis (see Chapter 4, page 88).

- **Figure 7.4**. A pneumothorax is not evident but there is air in the mediastinum and in the soft tissues of the neck. This was a complication of acute severe asthma but oesophageal perforation should be considered as well.

- **Figure 7.5**. The clue to the diagnosis is the peripheral distribution of the consolidation. This is an example of eosinophilic pneumonia, which responded promptly to corticosteroid therapy.

- **Figure 7.6**. A ring of calcium can be seen behind the heart and this is the left atrial wall, which has become calcified in response to long-standing elevation in left atrial pressure as a result of mitral stenosis. There are left-sided rib changes compatible with a left lateral thoracotomy and this woman had undergone a closed mitral valvotomy prior to her median sternotomy several years later (note the wire sternal sutures) and mitral valve replacement with a Starr-Edwards prosthesis (clearly seen) several years later.

- **Figure 7.7**. There is a 'white-out' of the left lung with some mediastinal shift to the opposite side – evidence of a large pleural effusion. A diagnostic pleural tap produced pus, and an intercostal drain was inserted into this massive empyema. Formal surgical drainage was subsequently required.

- **Figure 7.8**. There are multiple 'blotchy' shadows, linear shadows, toothpaste shadows and occasional tramlines, all in association with some cystic spaces. This combination of abnormalities is highly suggestive of bronchiectasis and this young person had cystic fibrosis.

- **Figure 7.9**. The differential diagnosis of superior mediastinal masses has been discussed in Chapter 2. Mediastinoscopy and biopsy in this case revealed Hodgkin's disease. Chest discomfort with alcohol is a well-described phenomenon in this situation.

- **Figure 7.10**. This shows extensive consolidation in the right lung with loss of volume in the very dense right upper lobe. Cavitation can be seen within the consolidation on the right and there are also a few fluffy shadows at the left apex. The combination of bilateral consolidation with loss of volume and cavitation is highly suggestive of tuberculosis – the diagnosis in this case.

- **Figure 7.11**. Sarcoidosis is suggested by the combination of bilateral hilar lymphadenopathy and the subtle, nodular, pulmonary infiltrate. The patient presented with painful ankles and erythema nodosum.

- **Figure 7.12**. There is dense consolidation within the right middle lobe (*Legionella* was the responsible organism) but this man's right arm is missing and there are sternal wires indicative of a previous sternotomy. An earlier motor-bike accident had been responsible for avulsion of the right arm and open chest surgery had been required in order to achieve haemostasis.

- **Figures 7.13 and 7.14**. Both films show evidence of nipple piercing. There is fairly generalized, bilateral consolidation in Fig. 7.13 and the obvious abnormality in Fig. 7.14 is the large ring-shadow in the right upper zone containing a fluid level. *Pneumocystis* pneumonia and lung abscess are the respective diagnoses and the common pathology was human immunodeficiency virus (HIV) infection in two intravenous drug abusers.

- **Figure 7.15**. The pulmonary infiltrate consists of tiny nodules distributed throughout the lung fields and extending even to the apices. This elderly Indian woman had miliary tuberculosis. This is the commonest explanation for this particular infiltrate but other possible diagnoses include micronodular metastases and sarcoidosis.

- **Figure 7.16**. There is an extensive bilateral pulmonary infiltrate, which seems to be composed of nodules but confluent in large areas. The differential diagnosis is wide and includes infection, malignancy, granulomatous infiltrate, interstitial pulmonary fibrosis and pulmonary haemorrhage. In fact, this was an example of acute extrinsic allergic alveolitis – 'bird-fancier's lung'.

- **Figure 7.17**. This pulmonary infiltrate is quite clearly nodular and some of the nodules are quite large. Heart size is normal and there is no evidence for associated lymph node, pleural or bony disease. Once again, the differential diagnosis is broad – this was chickenpox pneumonia in a young adult who was in respiratory failure and required assisted ventilation for more than a week.

- **Figure 7.18**. There are large areas of confluent consolidation throughout both lung fields. The margins of the abnormal shadowing are indistinct and are interspersed with 'streaky', linear shadows that suggest fibrotic change. This combination of appearances is odd, not looking like typical infection or malignant infiltration (although both are possible). Vasculitis, some form of interstitial fibrosis or extrinsic allergic alveolitis all figure in the differential diagnosis. This was a drug-induced pulmonary infiltrate – amiodarone lung.

- **Figure 7.19**. There is extensive, bilateral calcification, which is typically pleural in nature. The differential diagnosis of pleural calcification is old tuberculous empyema, calcified asbestos plaques and previous pleural haemorrhage. The shadowing is far too extensive to be organized pleural haemorrhage and the diagnostic 'give-aways' are the characteristic lace-work pleural pattern (the 'holly-leaf' pattern) and the linear calcification on the hemidiaphragms. These are asbestos pleural plaques – 'pattern recognition'!

- **Figure 7.20**. As mentioned, the most obvious abnormality is the extensive shadowing behind the heart in the left lower lobe associated with a pleural effusion. Unfortunately, this proved to be a bronchial carcinoma. Comprehensive observation (including the 'Four Bs') will also detect that the trachea is indented and shifted to the left by a right paratracheal mass that contains a rounded calcified shadow. This was a retrosternal thyroid goitre containing a calcified thyroid adenoma, quite unrelated to the bronchial carcinoma.

- **Figure 7.21**. There is a large, thick-walled shadow at the base of the left lung, which contains an air–fluid interface. It is possible that this is intrapulmonary, representing a lung abscess or cavitating carcinoma or infarct perhaps, but the appearances are more in keeping with pleural pathology. Computed tomography (CT) scanning would differentiate these two possibilities. The presence of both air and fluid in the pleural space can be explained by a broncho-pleural fistula, previous instrumentation of the pleural space (tapping or drainage) that has allowed air to enter from outside the chest wall, or vanishingly rarely, empyema due to a gas-forming organism. This was an empyema that had been incompletely drained. Management hinges on complete drainage and surgical intervention may be necessary as was the case with this patient.

- **Figure 7.22**. The perihilar infiltrate most resembles an alveolar-filling pattern. One cannot be certain of heart size on this AP film, nor can we see interstitial lines but there is some blunting of the left costo-phrenic angle (possible effusion) and heart failure seems a likely possibility. The perceptive will also have noticed the line shadow extending from right apex to upper border of the right hilum – the typical appearance of an azygos fissure. Finally, there are metal clips in the superior mediastinum indicative of previous mediastinal surgery, in this case removal of a retrosternal goitre.

- **Figure 7.23**. There is a huge amount of air under both hemidiaphragms. This elderly woman presented with an acute abdomen secondary to perforation of a colonic diverticulum. There is also clear evidence of old tuberculosis with bilateral calcified hilar glands and nodules of calcium in the right apex. Finally, the right shoulder is grossly disrupted – possibly due to rheumatoid arthritis.

- **Figure 7.24**. The lung fields appear hyper-inflated, the diaphragms are flat and the chest wall is hyper-expanded. This is a radiograph of a patient with extremely severe asthma. Overlying the left base (probably in a shirt pocket) is the outline of an aerosol inhaler, which looks empty. This was indeed a salbutamol inhaler and it was empty as a result of repeated use before medical help arrived.

- **Figure 7.25**. This is the X-ray of an older woman, showing calcium within the aortic arch and also in costochondral cartilages. Remember the 'four B's' (in this case, 'below the diaphragms') because there is also a calcified ring shadow below the left hemidiaphragm. This was thought to be a calcified splenic cyst. None of these appearances is of any great relevance.

- **Figure 7.26**. Apologies for the clue because this was a gunshot wound. The bullet can be seen very close to the left heart border and is associated with air-space shadowing secondary to traumatic haemorrhage.

FASCINOMAS

Here are some unusual chest X-rays that I have encountered over the years.

Figures 7.27 and 7.28

These are two examples of 'plombage' – a long-extinct surgical technique for the treatment of tuberculosis. In Fig. 7.27, multiple dense rings can be seen at the left apex and similar shadows are bilateral in Fig. 7.28. Spheres of an early plastic, called leucite, were inserted into the pleural cavity in an attempt to create permanent localized collapse of lung infected with tuberculosis (scattered dots of intrapulmonary calcification, indicative of old tuberculosis, can be seen in the right upper zone in Fig. 7.28) because *Mycobacterium tuberculosis* is an organism that does not tolerate poor ventilation.

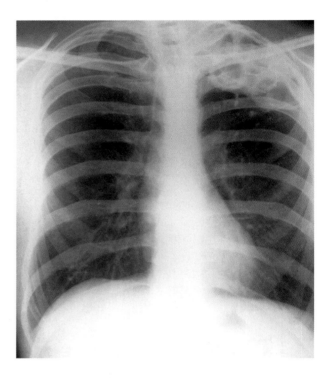

Figure 7.27 See text.

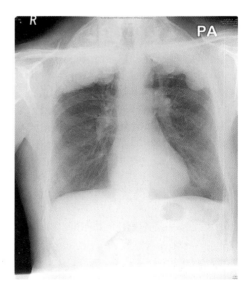

Figure 7.28 See text.

Figures 7.29 and 7.30

These are the postero-anterior (PA) and lateral chest X-rays of a child who was the son of a sheep farmer in west Wales. Note the 'halo' sign within the mass, seen particularly well in the lateral view. This was an intrapulmonary hydatid cyst.

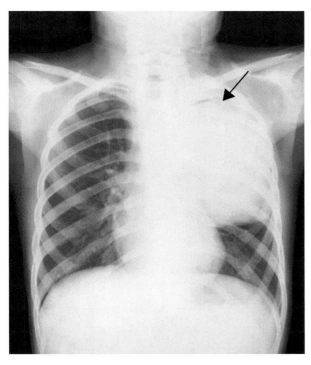

Figure 7.29 See text.

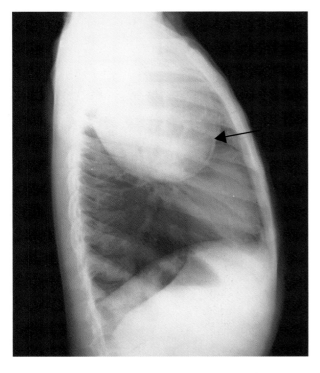

Figure 7.30 See text.

Figures 7.31 and 7.32

A 30-year-old Indonesian sailor docked in Cardiff in the late 1970s and promptly attended the Cardiff Chest Clinic complaining of weight loss and haemoptysis. Subtle ring shadows could just be seen in the right mid-zone on his radiograph but these do not reproduce well here. Dr Brian Davies (my boss at the time) made the stunning diagnosis of paragonimiasis on the basis of the history and the patient's ethnic background. He was absolutely correct and the bronchogram (Fig. 7.32) shows saccules representing the burrows of the lung fluke. *Paragonimus* has a complicated life cycle, which involves a freshwater snail, shell-fish and human hosts at different stages. Humans usually become infected by eating raw shell-fish. In Indonesia, there is a favoured dish called 'drunken crab' (raw crab marinated in alcohol) and this appeared to be the source of infection in this case.

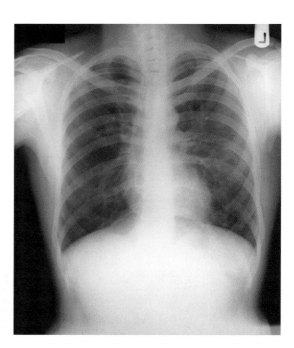

Figure 7.31 See text.

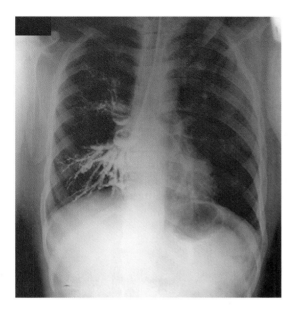

Figure 7.32 See text.

Figure 7.33

Right paratracheal lymphadenopathy can be seen in this X-ray of a young child. This was a manifestation of primary pulmonary tuberculosis. Note the mediastinal shift to the left, which was accompanied by obstructive emphysema of the right lung. These mechanical changes occurred due to partial collapse of immature airways as a result of extrinsic compression.

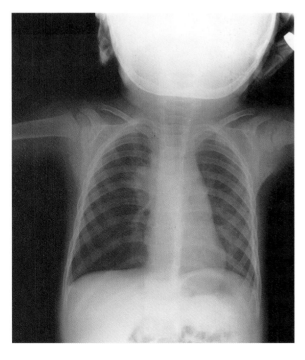

Figure 7.33 See text.

Figure 7.34

This man had worked as a coal miner in eastern Germany under appalling conditions for some years until he migrated to this country in 1950. He then worked at the Nottinghamshire coal-face and had a series of chest X-rays taken from the early 1960s until this film, dating from 1978. The earlier films showed faint intrapulmonary nodulation, which calcified progressively over the years. Despite the striking X-ray appearances, his functional disability was relatively slight and the diagnosis had always been a puzzle – the slow calcification and the nature of the shadows not really fitting with any clear diagnosis. There was, of course, an assumption that the radiographic changes were related in some way to his industrial exposure, but the changes were in no way like silicosis and a negative rheumatoid factor made an unusual example of Caplan's syndrome untenable. The diagnosis of extensive intrapulmonary amyloidosis was finally made at post mortem, following a fatal myocardial infarction.

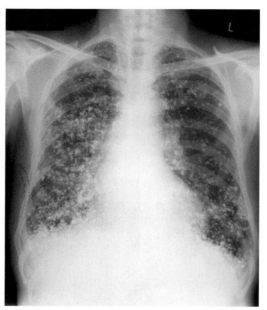

Figure 7.34 See text.

Figures 7.35 and 7.36

This woman was referred for biopsy of the intrapulmonary nodule seen lying just within the left heart border on the PA X-ray. However, careful radiographic examination revealed several other subtle intrapulmonary nodules (right mid-zone in Fig. 7.35) and, on clinical examination, she had telangiectasia on her lips. The pulmonary angiogram (Fig. 7.36) shows multiple arteriovenous malformations, which are recognized associations of the Osler–Rendu–Weber syndrome.

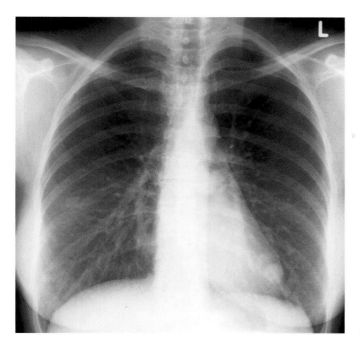

Figure 7.35 See text.

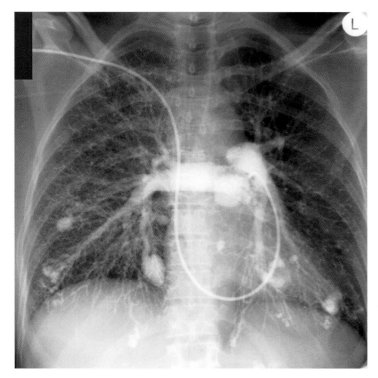

Figure 7.36 See text.

IN CONCLUSION

I think this case is an appropriate way to conclude the chapter and the book. It emphasizes the need for systematic, thorough chest X–ray interpretation as well as the importance of combining clinical and radiographic information when caring for individual patients.

Many of the skills of clinical medicine are generic and, when interpreting a chest X-ray, adopt a problem-solving, 'detective's' approach. Be disciplined and systematic in your observations and glean as much information from the radiograph as possible. Be wary of diagnostic and management pitfalls, and the book has highlighted a variety of these. Finally, if in any doubt, seek help.

Index

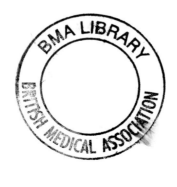